100 Questions & Answers About Life After Cancer: A Survivor's Guide

Page Tolbert, LCSW

The Post-Treatment Resource Program
Memorial Sloan-Kettering Cancer Center
New York, NY

Penny Damaskos, LCSW, OSWC

The Post-Treatment Resource Program
Memorial Sloan-Kettering Cancer Center
New York, NY

JONES AND BARTLETT PUBLISHERS
Sudbury, Massachusetts
BOSTON   TORONTO   LONDON   SINGAPORE

World Headquarters
Jones and Bartlett Publishers
40 Tall Pine Drive
Sudbury, MA 01776
978-443-5000
info@jbpub.com
www.jbpub.com

Jones and Bartlett Publishers
Canada
6339 Ormindale Way
Mississauga, Ontario L5V 1J2
CANADA

Jones and Bartlett Publishers
International
Barb House, Barb Mews
London W6 7PA
UK

Jones and Bartlett's books and products are available through most bookstores and online booksellers. To contact Jones and Bartlett Publishers directly, call 800-832-0034, fax 978-443-8000, or visit our website, www.jbpub.com.

Substantial discounts on bulk quantities of Jones and Bartlett's publications are available to corporations, professional associations, and other qualified organizations. For details and specific discount information, contact the special sales department at Jones and Bartlett via the above contact information or send an email to specialsales@jbpub.com.

The authors, editor, and publisher have made every effort to provide accurate information. However, they are not responsible for errors, omissions, or for any outcomes related to the use of the contents of this book and take no responsibility for the use of the products and procedures described. Treatments and side effects described in this book may not be applicable to all people; likewise, some people may require a dose or experience a side effect that is not described herein. Drugs and medical devices are discussed that may have limited availability controlled by the Food and Drug Administration (FDA) for use only in a research study or clinical trial. Research, clinical practice, and government regulations often change the accepted standard in this field. When consideration is being given to use of any drug in the clinical setting, the health care provider or reader is responsible for determining FDA status of the drug, reading the package insert, and reviewing prescribing information for the most up-to-date recommendations on dose, precautions, and contraindications, and determining the appropriate usage for the product. This is especially important in the case of drugs that are new or seldom used.

Production Credits
Executive Publisher: Christopher Davis
Production Director: Amy Rose
Associate Editor: Kathy Richardson
Production Assistant: Leah Corrigan
V.P., Manufacturing and Inventory Control:
   Therese Connell
Associate Marketing Manager: Rebecca Wasley

Composition: Appingo
Cover Design: Jonathan Ayotte
Printing and Binding: Malloy, Inc.
Cover Printing: Malloy, Inc.
Cover Images: ©Yuri Arcurs/ShutterStock, Inc.,
   ©Galina Barskaya/ShutterStock, Inc.,
   ©Kirk Peart Professional Imaging/
   ShutterStock, Inc.

Library of Congress Cataloging-in-Publication Data
Tolbert, Page.
  100 questions and answers about life after cancer : a survivor's guide / Page Tolbert and Penny Damaskos.
    p. cm.
Includes index.
  ISBN 978-0-7637-5069-5 (alk. paper)
  1. Cancer--Miscellanea. 2. Cancer--Patients--Life skills guides. I. Damaskos, Penny. II. Title. III. Title: One hundred questions and answers about life after cancer.
  RC263.T65 2008
  616.99'4--dc22
  6048   2007025866
Printed in the United States of America
11 10 09 08 07   10 9 8 7 6 5 4 3 2 1

To Jim and Julie, with gratitude and love.

CONTENTS

Foreword   ix

Preface   xi

Acknowledgments   xiii

Introduction   xv

Part 1: Survivorship: A Mixed Blessing   1

Questions 1–17 cover the complex feelings that come with finishing treatment:
- When should I consider myself a survivor?
- Why do I have mixed feelings about finishing treatment?
- Could I be depressed?

Part 2: Managing Uncertainty   23

Questions 18–27 discuss the challenge of tolerating unanswered questions about the present and future:
- Why do I think it's cancer every time I have a headache?
- How do I cope with frightening statistics?
- Why do follow up appointments make me so upset?

Part 3: Communicating with Family and Friends   37

Questions 28–46 explore the complex reactions of those around you:
- Should I tell my friend that I've been hurt by her response to my illness?
- Why do people say such insensitive things?
- How do I let the people in my life know that I've changed since my cancer experience?

Part 4: Legal, Financial, and Workplace Concerns   63

Questions 47–64 outline your rights as a cancer survivor under the law, and discuss issues such as insurance and debt:
- Can my company fire me for being out sick?
- Can I get life insurance now that I have had cancer?
- What do I do about the debt I incurred while sick?

Part 5: Too Young for Cancer   85

Questions 65–68 address the special concerns of those who had cancer as children or young adults:
- Do I need to tell my new doctor of my childhood cancer? Why is it still important?
- I feel like such a baby since I moved back home with my parents during my treatment. Will I ever "catch up"?
- How do I deal with others my age who have never been sick and just don't get it?

Part 6: Maintaining Your Health   93

Questions 69–77 help to sort through the confused messages you may get about staying healthy:
- Is a "positive attitude" important?
- What about diet?
- Will stress make me get sick again?

Part 7: Sex, Intimacy, and Fertility   105

Questions 78–89 cover concerns about reconnecting with your partner, or connecting with a new one, and address feelings about your changed body:
- Why is my partner avoiding me? Has she stopped caring?
- When do I tell someone I'm dating that I had cancer?
- My treatment caused me to become infertile. How do I deal with this loss?

Part 8: Growth, Change, and Spirituality   123

Questions 90–94 address the new and different feelings you may have about who you are after cancer:
- I used to have a strong religious faith, but feel I've lost it since cancer. Will I ever get it back?
- Some survivors tell me that they gained a lot from their cancer experience. Can this be true?
- Is there something wrong with me if I don't make big changes after cancer?

Part 9: Cancer as a Chronic Illness   133

Questions 95–100 discuss what it is like to live with cancer, rather than beyond it:
- If I have metastatic illness, does that mean I'm not a survivor?
- My disease has recurred. Does that mean I've failed?
- My doctor says there is no further treatment for my illness. If I can't be cured, is there any help available for me?

Appendix   141

A list of resources and websites that offer advice and
guidance on many aspects of survivorship.

Glossary   155

Index   159

Contents

It is remarkable that there are now 10 million cancer survivors in the United States today. What a wonderful contrast to 30 years ago when the term "cancer survivor" was quite new. As one who has lived through this era in cancer medicine, it is gratifying to see the concern now for this large group of people who have survived cancer—and whose issues are being carefully addressed. I recall when patients who reported problems after cancer treatment were told, "Just be thankful you are alive, and don't complain." Happily, those days are over, and the range of survivors' issues are being given attention.

I can think of no two people better equipped to write a book for survivors than these two authors who have been on the "front line" of survivorship in the Post-Treatment Resource Program of Memorial Sloan-Kettering Cancer Center. This was one of the very first such programs to provide crucial information for those early survivors about their psychological and social problems in the 1980s, addressing issues about jobs, legal rights, and how to manage talking with friends and colleagues.

The format of questions and answers is excellent, and the reader who is interested in the range of issues for survivors of cancer will find this very much to their liking and their needs.

Jimmie Holland, MD
Attending Psychiatrist
Wayne E. Chapman Chair in Psychiatric Oncology
Memorial Sloan-Kettering Cancer Center
New York, NY

Our years of working with patients have taught us that cancer brings with it one crisis after another. The shock of diagnosis is soon followed by the anxiety and fear that come with the beginning of treatment. Whether a person has to undergo surgery, radiation, chemotherapy, or a combination of these modalities, starting on a passage through such uncharted territory can be daunting. But once the treatment is over, another journey begins. This is the journey through survivorship.

Many patients are stunned to learn that the very outcome they have most hoped for brings with it new challenges. Most feel deeply changed by their cancer experience, and enter survivorship feeling disoriented by this sense of "differentness." In our work, we have seen time and again that many of the shifts that take place are profoundly positive. But what we've learned, too, is that even positive change takes getting used to.

While no two cancer survivors are the same, many of their questions echo each other: How do I cope with new and different priorities? Why don't friends and family understand what I feel? What about discrimination in the workplace? This book provides answers to these questions, as well as others that we have heard through the years. We intend it to serve as a guide through the new, and sometimes confusing, world of life after cancer.

Page Tolbert, LCSW
Penny Damaskos, LCSW

ACKNOWLEDGMENTS

We would like to thank both the professionals (nurses, doctors, social workers, and others) and the "experts" (survivors) who contributed to this project. This book would not have been possible without the help of the following mentors, colleagues, and contributors:

Jane Bowling, DSW; Mary McCabe, RN, MA; Jimmie Holland, MD; Kevin Oeffinger, MD; Nancy Houlihan, RN, MA, AOCN; Roz Kleban, LCSW; Tara Leflein, LCSW; Beth Whittam, RN, CFNP; Jane Mather, MA, NACC; Donald Garrity, RD, CDN; Randye Retkin, Esq.; David McDaniel, Esq.; Jane Hedal-Siegel; Clarissa Potter, LCSW; Rachel Schneider, LCSW; Karrie Zampini, LCSW; Stephanie Stratigos; and last but not least, Susanne, Angela, Brian, Judy, and Dave.

We owe our thanks to our wise, generous, and supportive colleagues too numerous to mention and, of course, to our legions of survivors who have taught us so much over the years and who continue to do so.

Today we can celebrate the over 10 million Americans who have survived their cancer, a number unimaginable 25 or 30 years ago. This history-making group includes people decades beyond their diagnosis, which reflects the great strides and advances in cancer research and treatment. Daily, new survivors are being added to the ranks of this growing population as survival rates for most cancers continue to improve. Along with this great news, though, it is important for us to remember that there are complex underlying themes experienced by cancer survivors—parallel feelings of gratitude and confusion or uncertainty, worry as well as joy, and sometimes a deep sense of aloneness or isolation. Wellness is one thing, but well-being another.

Journeying through and beyond the cancer experience can be confusing to the survivor and the health care provider alike. Many questions arise. "My friends and family are so glad my cancer is 'over.' Why don't I feel like it is?" or "My friends and family tell me that the cancer is in the past, and I should forget it now that I'm well. But somehow I don't want to do that. Does this mean I'm dwelling on a negative experience?" In my experience working with cancer survivors of all ages, these are typical questions expressed by my patients as they seek to blend their cancer experience with their precancer life and seek understanding and context.

Where should a survivor look for more information to help answer these questions? In our internet-age of information overload, there is much out there, but is it reliable; is it trustworthy? What resources can a health care provider suggest to his or her patients?

Page Tolbert and Penny Damaskos have devoted their careers to working with cancer survivors. Indeed, between the two of them, they have 35 years of experience in this area. Over the years, they have developed innumerable resources that we health care providers depend upon. Time and time again, they have provided immeasurable help to our cancer survivors, hearing their fears and concerns, counseling with them, and helping to smooth out the bumps and potholes in the survivor experience. And now they share from their rich and meaningful experiences in crafting this wonderful book, *100 Questions and Answers About Life After Cancer: A Survivor's Guide.*

This book reflects what my patients ask at their clinic visits, what their spouses or partners share with me, what their mothers call about, what their children are worried about. Their very thoughtful and salient responses to these questions will provide meaning, context, direction, and validation for much of what cancer survivors and their families experience. And most importantly, their guidance is trustworthy and invaluable. I hope that this book becomes a starting point for all cancer survivors.

Those of us who follow and care for cancer survivors will find this book a necessity—in fact, it should be required reading for all who deal with cancer survivors. I hope and anticipate that we as health care professionals will point our patients to this wonderful resource, and then reflect with them as they struggle to put their cancer experience into context.

Kevin C. Oeffinger, MD
*Director, Program for Adult Survivors of
Pediatric Cancer
Departments of Pediatrics and Medicine
Memorial Sloan-Kettering Cancer Center
New York, NY*

PART ONE

Survivorship: A Mixed Blessing

When should I consider myself a cancer survivor?

I'm confused. Should I say, "I have cancer," or "I had cancer?"

I couldn't wait for treatment to be finished. Why do I have mixed feelings now that it's over?

More . . .

1. When should I consider myself a cancer survivor? Do I start counting from the date I was diagnosed, or the date my treatment ended?

This question is definitely one of the most pressing for people who have been treated for cancer. Finding an answer, however, can be frustrating because the response may differ depending on whom you ask. One doctor might tell you to count from the date of diagnosis, another from the end of treatment, and a third may say that such a process of counting is meaningless. What this lack of consensus really tells us is that there is no clear "cancer clock." We believe that one reason people are so eager for clarity on this issue is that they have heard that there is a certain point at which they can consider themselves cured of their disease. It is understandable that a survivor would want to know when she can breathe easy and stop worrying about recurrence. In many cases she has heard the media refer to a five-year cutoff point, and so she is anxiously waiting for that date to arrive.

But in the real world, the answer isn't that simple. It may be that the figure of five years came about because many studies refer to the "five-year survival rate" of various illnesses. But each cancer is different. For some, being five years down the road does indeed mean that your cancer is unlikely to recur; in other cases it means very little. In still others, such as some forms of thyroid cancer, your doctor may tell you that you're cured the minute you awaken from surgery.

Again, it's only natural to want a timetable for full recovery. But sometimes focusing on this goal robs you of enjoying your life in the moment. If at all possible, try to focus on the present, and try to make the most of every day—rather than counting them.

2. I'm confused. Should I say, "I have cancer," or "I had cancer?"

If you had the flu and then recovered, you wouldn't say "I have the flu." So why do so many cancer survivors ask this question? We think it may be because the cancer experience is unique in so many ways.

In many instances people don't know they have cancer until a test or scan reveals that this is the case. It's understandable that, if you could have a disease without knowing it was there, you might *still* have that disease, and not know about it. Naturally, if you have undergone the recommended treatment and your doctor tells you that you are disease-free, there is every reason to believe you are. If you have doubts, ask your doctor how he knows that you are now free of cancer.

Additionally, there are people who are so fearful that their cancer will return that they can't move into "survivorship mode." It feels safer to just say "I have cancer, and always will." This stance doesn't reflect their true medical status. In this case, some counseling about their anxiety may be helpful.

Another reason we think this question crops up, is that cancer can be an identity-altering experience. Many patients vividly describe the feeling of moving from one world—the world of the well—into another—the world of illness—when they receive their diagnosis. They go from feeling like healthy, normal people to feeling "different." Turning this way of thinking around doesn't happen instantly, just because your doctor says you are well. Most people do feel changed by their cancer experience, and, in fact, many *want* to acknowledge that change. There are some survivors who tell us that they will always be a "cancer person," even as they move past their diagnosis and treatment, and not all of them

Most people feel changed by their cancer experience and want to acknowledge this change.

are sad or distressed by this; some are even proud of having faced a challenge and survived.

But remember—if your health care team tells you that you are cancer-free, there is no reason not to believe that this is the case.

3. I couldn't wait for treatment to be finished. Why do I have mixed feelings now that it's over?

It has to be confusing to go through something as hard as treatment for cancer and not feel 100% happy when it's over. And yet, if we had to name the question most frequently asked by people finishing treatment, it would be this one.

It's natural for you, and those around you, to think that the end of this challenging and stressful time will bring nothing but relief. And yet, for many new survivors, this isn't the case. Instead, they often describe feeling "adrift," "cut off" or "on my own." After months of being cared for and monitored by your health care team, you suddenly stop being in such close touch with them. Let's let Marty, an oral cancer survivor describe it:

For weeks, I saw my radiation tech every day. Even though I didn't like going for treatments, I always liked chatting with Debbie. She answered my questions, and her warm smile always made me feel better. Now I won't be seeing her, and, after all this time, it feels strange.

Chemotherapy

The use of drugs to treat cancer throughout the body.

Radiation

Use of x-rays to shrink tumors and kill cancerous cells.

In addition to missing the security and reassurance provided by your team, the end of **chemotherapy** or **radiation** can be hard for other reasons. As Lydia, a breast cancer survivor put it:

While I was on chemo, I felt like I was doing something—fighting back against the cancer. Now I feel unprotected—like my disease will come back if I don't keep taking treatment.

Laurie, a survivor of ovarian cancer went even further:

I would be willing to be on chemo the rest of my life, if it would keep the cancer away!

Many people say that they are genuinely relieved to complete their treatment. But in addition to those positive feelings, they may also have the sense of aloneness and vulnerability described by Marty and Lydia. These mixed feelings are a natural part of the transition from active treatment, and are to be expected. They don't mean you are ungrateful to be finished—or that, like Laurie, you actually wish you could have another round of chemo! But they do tell us that being a cancer survivor brings its own challenges. It can be a difficult adjustment to lose the constant scrutiny and support that you've had since your diagnosis. Sometimes people even describe feeling superstitious about their disease returning if their doctors and nurses aren't there to "keep it away." But it's important to remember that there is a right time for treatment to end. When your regimen is complete, it means your team feels that you've had the appropriate dose of chemotherapy or radiation. This opinion has been formed over a long period of time, and is the result of much study and experimentation. So, let yourself experience all the feelings that come with the end of treatment, and know that you're not alone. But know, too, that you've had the amount of treatment that your doctor thinks is best, and you're not moving forward without the protection that that offers.

Angela, a 43-year-old survivor of Hodgkin's disease, comments:

Now that it's over. Well, from my perspective it never really is over. "Over" implies that you go back to where you were before. But the experience of cancer and its treatment changes you forever. It changes how you see your life, the world around you, your relationships with others, your relationship with your body, and the way you make decisions for the rest of your life. It is forever part of your story.

Many people miss the security provided by frequent contact with their health care team.

At first you are scared of being cut off from the people who helped you get better. And that includes family and friends. Cancer organizes your life. Gives you a mission and a plan. It focuses everything for a while. Losing that sense of mission and getting on with your life is very, very scary. The fear of relapse is intense and plays out in all sorts of conscious and unconscious ways. Over time I have come to see this fear as a lifelong irritating companion. Much like the tinnitus that I was left with after my BMT, the fear is at times louder than others. It tends to pop up when I have big decisions to make or big changes are afoot. It took me and my loved ones a long time to realize that the fear never really goes away. For me, the one place I can continue to face that fear, handle it, manage it, and stash it back in its place is with continued intermittent psychotherapy.

The fear of relapse is very, very real. Especially for those, like me, who have had one. I try to go to the doctor whenever I have a concern or fear. I'm religious about annual exams and I'm lucky to have a doctor who monitors me carefully.

4. My friends and family are so glad my cancer is "over." Why don't I feel like it is?

Your friends and family care for you and want you to be well. It's understandable that they would want to think of your cancer experience as being in the past. You would probably like that, too. But the experience of cancer doesn't end with your last radiation treatment or with your doctor's handshake of congratulations. As we have discussed previously, you can't go through diagnosis and treatment without having some sort of reaction; if you didn't, you wouldn't be human. Chances are, you are still reflecting on the news that you have cancer, as well as recalling the distress and disruption of treatment. You may also have some of the feelings that other survivors described earlier—of being unsafe or unprotected—now that treatment is completed. Many new survivors describe fear of recurrence as their number one concern. They may become much more aware of every bodily sensation and spend a great deal of time worrying about their health. With all of this going on, it is unlikely that you would view your cancer as being "over."

Try to understand why those around you may pressure you to put your cancer in the past before you are ready to do so. This may actually come from their concern for you, and perhaps from the anxiety that your cancer diagnosis has raised about their own health. But you can also tell them that your recovery begins now, and that it is an ongoing process without a clear "end date."

Dave, a 63-year-old survivor of colorectal cancer, comments:

I think that keeping cancer awareness near the surface is helpful and reduces the stress that may come from avoiding the topic. My family is very close and they follow my post-treatment activities very closely. We discuss the follow-up in detail. I think this open approach is healthy, both for the family and me. I also post a family Web site and update after each follow-up appointment so that anyone interested can find the latest information. In this way, they remain aware that the battle with cancer is constant. We can never know the future, but we can maintain a watchful state and strictly adhere to the follow-up protocols. We may be cured, or we may be harboring a few latent cells that have the potential to recur. That uncertainty is really no different than anyone else's state in this world.

5. During my treatment, I did fine. Everyone agreed that I was a real trooper—my kids even called me a hero! Now I find that I'm sad; I even cry sometimes. Does this mean I'm weak?

A diagnosis of cancer is one of the most frightening events a person can experience. It's understandable that when you're told that you have a life-threatening illness, you want to do whatever it takes to treat that illness, and you want to do it ASAP. This is a time when many people set aside thoughts and emotions about cancer in order to do what their doctor recommends. They want to get going with treatment, so that they can be assured that they are doing all they can to eradicate the cancer. An unusual number of survivors have used the same phrase to describe being on treatment: "I just put one foot in front of the other." What they are describing is a state of mind that doesn't allow for reflection or strong emotion. Patients may literally set these feelings aside, in order to give all their attention to getting well. One patient said, "Being on treatment was like my army days, just follow orders and march!"

It's understandable that others admire what they see as stoicism and strength—and of course, those characteristics are part of getting through treatment, too. But when treatment ends, there is finally time to process all the feelings that one has set aside while "marching in step." This type of reaction doesn't apply only to cancer patients. Many survivors of combat or crime will also describe being calm and collected while going through the experience, but shaking or crying when it is over. This is the way that our body and psyche discharge strong emotion that has been held in check during a crisis. Far from being weak, it is an appropriate response to a life-threatening situation, which, after all, is what you have been through.

Letting out strong emotions after treatments ends is normal.

Try to go easy on yourself during this time. Letting out your emotions now is normal and may allow you to heal emotionally even faster than you would if you continued to keep them at bay. It may be hard for your family to see you upset, but you can tell them that this is what often happens to people when something very hard is over. They will still understand that you got through a big challenge, and will not lose their admiration for you. You can reassure them that you need this time to "let it all out," so that you can regain and refocus your energy on life as it continues after cancer.

6. My neighbor had cancer last year, and she says she never thinks about it now. But I think of my illness all the time. Does that mean she's braver than I am?

Once again, it's important to remember that each cancer survivor is an individual, and people will react to their illness in different ways. Comparing yourself to others is truly a case of apples and oranges, and can only cause stress. Your neighbor may be telling the truth about her experience, but she may also be coping with some of the painful or worrisome aspects of cancer survivorship by burying it somewhere inside. Sometimes this works, but it can also backfire. The experience of cancer always involves some level of loss—even if it's only the loss of your "healthy self." After a loss, it is necessary to grieve, just as you would if you lost an important person in your life. This grieving process is part of what allows us to discharge our pain and move on. Could it be that your neighbor has been trying to avoid this in some way? It could be that you are engaged in an important kind of mourning, which will eventually contribute to your growth and permit you to move to a place where you can reflect on your cancer experience with less distress and anxiety. Your neighbor may actually be missing out on something. But again, everyone is different, and her style of coping may be just right for her. In any case, don't compare your own healing to anyone else's. Remember, there is no one "right" way to respond.

7. My friends and family tell me that cancer is in the past and that I should forget it now that I'm well. But somehow I don't want to do that. Does this mean I'm dwelling on a negative experience?

As we've mentioned before, it's natural for the people in your life to want you to leave the distress and disruption of your cancer experience behind you. Your family cares for you, and

*It takes time
to sort out all
your feelings
about the cancer
experience;
don't rush
yourself.*

**Bone marrow
transplant,
allogeneic**

A medical procedure
in which healthy
stem cells are
donated by another
person (a donor),
who may or may
not be related to the
patient, but whose
cells must be a good
genetic match, and
given to the patient
after high-dose
chemotherapy;
sometimes used as
part of the treatment
for cancers that are
in the bone marrow,
such as leukemia and
multiple myeloma.

**Bone marrow
transplant,
autologous**

A medical procedure
in which cells are
obtained from one's
own bone marrow,
frozen, and reinfused
after high-dose
chemotherapy is
given.

wants to forget the pain that your cancer gave to all of you. Your friends may feel the same way. At work, your boss and colleagues may also be affected—some because they care for you and some because they want you to resume the tasks you performed before. People's wish for you to stop thinking or talking about cancer can add up to a lot of pressure, especially when they label you as "negative." But you don't need to give in to that pressure—and you probably couldn't do so anyway. The cancer experience can be overwhelming and may affect you in many ways. It takes time to sort out all the ways that you feel changed by your experience, and for each survivor the time needed is different. Of course, in some ways, your cancer experience will affect you throughout your lifetime by altering the way that you view the world. Clearly, you can't put such a powerful experience behind you overnight.

But you're also saying that you don't *want* to do that, and many survivors say that as well. It's important to them to "digest" their experience and learn from it. Doing so is not "negative," but is in fact *necessary* for their healing. This may be true no matter how painful or challenging that experience has been. As a matter of fact, the more painful an ordeal they have undergone (such as a **bone marrow transplant**), the more they may need to revisit and reflect on what they have been through. This is not the same as "dwelling" on something negative, which implies thinking only of one's misfortune and pain, over and over again, without its leading anywhere. (And let's be frank—if you wanted to do that for a while, it would be understandable, and is no one's business but yours!) As hard as it is, try not to let the judgments of others guide your recovery process.

A funny P.S. to this answer: One of our women's groups continued to meet once a month for many years, finding a warm and sustaining connection with each other. From time to time, one of them would be in touch, informing us that they had just had a "dwelling" last week, or that a "dwelling" was coming up. When finally questioned about this unusual name, one of them explained with a laugh, "That's what we call it, because our husbands keep saying 'Are you still dwelling on that?!'"

8. I was treated for breast cancer, and my doctor says I'm doing fine. But she has placed me on a hormonal treatment. Does this mean I'm still on treatment?

The short answer is yes. You are on treatment in the positive sense that your doctor is addressing the cancer you had, as well as working to prevent any cancer that might occur in the future. But the vast majority of people find that **hormonal treatment** is not as disruptive to their lives in the same way that chemotherapy or radiation can be. In most cases it permits them to pick up their usual activities, to look the way they used to, and to feel fairly normal. Many women choose to think of hormonal treatments as a kind of maintenance— something they do to stay well, rather than to get well.

Hormonal treatment

Treatment that blocks the effect of hormones in hormone-dependent cancers.

Over the past few years, hormonal treatment has been used more and more in addressing hormonally-related cancers, such as breast, ovarian, and prostate cancer. In many ways, hormonal medication has changed the face of treating these cancers, often presenting a less toxic alternative, which is still remarkably effective. There is now a wide variety of medications that come under this category. Obviously your doctor has made a decision about which one is most appropriate for you.

9. My treatment ended a year ago. Afterwards I felt sad, frightened about recurrence, and confused about who I was. Now I feel much better, but not 100%. Will I ever move beyond where I am?

After cancer, everyone moves forward on their own timetable.

After the cancer experience, everyone moves forward on their own timetable, so don't assume that you have come as far as you're going to go; your healing will continue. It's especially important not to compare yourself to others, or to "measure" your progress. The experience of cancer is powerful and affects so many parts of who you are; it's only natural for it to take some time to adjust to this new phase of your life. But that being said, it's also true that you're unlikely to ever feel exactly the same as you did before your diagnosis. One survivor put this eloquently. Pointing to a paperweight filled with a snow scene, she said, "My life is like that globe. It got shaken up, and when the storm stopped, all the same flakes were there—but they were all in a different place." This woman captured the feeling that many survivors have about all the ways that life may be different. Relationships may undergo change, with some people drawing nearer and others pulling back. Your world may also feel different because your own priorities have shifted; there are some people and activities that seem more important to you, and others that feel less so. It takes time for all of this to shake out, so be sure to go easy on yourself, and allow the time you need. Finally, it is true that some sadness about your experience of illness, and the changes that accompany it, may linger. But they will not necessarily get in the way of your emotional healing, and they may even add depth to your life. Only time will tell—so give yourself that time.

10. Everyone I know says "You look great!" I know they're trying to be nice—so why does this bother me so much?

This is an issue that arises repeatedly in our survivorship groups, so why don't we let the survivors respond first?

Lily: *I hate when people tell me how good I look! I still feel exhausted, and sometimes downright depressed. They're only seeing the outside, and obviously don't care about my real feelings.*

Karen: *I feel like they're pressuring me, like they're saying 'OK—you look fine, so the cancer's all over. Time to get back to normal.'*

Laurie: *Ha! I feel like they're saying 'I thought you were dead, but you look pretty good, so I guess you're not.'*

Arnie: *I feel negated by them! Like they don't recognize everything I have gone through! Sometimes people can be so blind.*

As you can see, survivors hear this in many different ways, and all of them may have an element of reality.

It's understandable that when you're feeling uncertain or sad on the inside, a compliment on the outside sounds superficial or even insensitive. Some survivors also feel so changed by their treatment—perhaps suffering hair loss, weight gain, or other problems—that a compliment feels meaningless at best, and insincere at worst. But it's important to ask yourself if you're projecting some of your own feelings on others—if *you're* feeling fat, bloated, and bald, then you're sure others see you that way, too. If you're exhausted, you can't believe it isn't evident to others. But that having been said, it may be very true that this simple question reflects multiple motivations. Most survivors find that, unless they have a reason to believe they are truly being insulted, a simple "thank you" is the best response. You can always add your own twist: "Thanks—more importantly, I feel good," or "Thanks, but looks are deceiving, I'm still pretty bushed."

11. I told my doctor that I feel down a lot thinking about my illness and that I cry very often. I also seem to wake up very early in the morning, and I can't get back to sleep. She diagnosed me as having depression and wants to prescribe medication to help. I was shocked! I feel like she's saying I have some kind of psychological problem, or that there's something wrong with me. Isn't she?

Depression may be one response to what you've been through; treatment can help.

It's easy to understand why you might be puzzled or even offended by what your doctor said. After all, cancer is a real problem, so feeling sad afterward is a natural and human response—not a psychological disorder; however, sometimes when we're very sad about something, especially over a long period of time, the chemistry of our brain actually changes, and this is where medication can make a difference. It should be noted that some cancer treatments themselves can actually cause **depression**, so be sure to ask your medical team about that.

Depression, clinical

An emotional disorder characterized by feelings of sadness, loss of appetite, insomnia, and inability to concentrate, often involving changes in brain chemistry.

Neurotransmitters

Chemicals made by brain cells to help "communicate" with another cell.

I don't understand. A pill can't erase the fact that I had cancer, or that I was passed over for a promotion at work, or that my wife and I seem to be snapping at each other. Since I have real problems, how can a medication help?

That is all true; there's not a pill in the world that can make painful experiences disappear, or make you happy that you had cancer! The chemical changes we mentioned, however, can make it harder for you to cope with the very real problems you face. Depression can cause your brain to reduce production of chemicals, called **neurotransmitters**, which help nerve cells to "speak" to each other. When these chemicals are not helping cells to communicate, you may feel sad, hopeless, tearful, and suffer from what doctors call "**psycho-motor retardation**," or a kind of slowing down. One woman described this feeling as "swimming through molasses." Again, it is not that your sad feelings don't have a basis in reality, only that they may set off chemical changes that can make you feel worse. In depression, the neurotransmitter whose production is disrupted most frequently is **serotonin**. It may be that the brain lacks the chemical material to make serotonin, that there is not enough serotonin being produced, or that your brain lacks the sites to receive and use this important substance. **Dopamine** and **norepinephrine** are other brain chemicals which may affect mood in some individuals. Medication can correct the imbalance in these neurotransmitters and get you back on the road to feeling better. In addition to improving your mood, **antidepressant medication** may also increase your ability to concentrate, give a small boost to your energy level, or even help relieve some types of chronic pain. It's unlikely that your doctor will recommend that you remain on such medication for a long time—just long enough to get you past this difficult period.

12. But won't I become dependent on medication to feel good? I want to be able to make it on my own, and medicine sounds like a crutch to me.

The medication given for depression is not **addictive**. And as far as being a crutch goes, if you had a headache, would you consider aspirin a crutch? Would you blame a diabetic, whose body chemistry is also altered, for taking insulin? Probably not. There are many aspects to depression, but one of those aspects is the very real chemical changes described previously; antidepressant medication is designed specifically to address this altered chemistry.

Psycho-motor retardation

Slowing down of movement and thinking, often found in those with clinical depression.

Serotonin

A neurotransmitter created in the central nervous system, often associated with feelings of well-being.

Dopamine

A neurotransmitter in the central nervous system that regulates emotion and movement.

Norepinephrine

A neurotransmitter in the central nervous system, connected with the "fight or flight" response, as well as reaction to stress.

Antidepressant medication

Drugs used to alleviate the symptoms of clinical depression, such as sadness, insomnia, and lack of energy.

Addictive

Describing something that is physically or psychologically habit-forming, so that discontinuation causes extreme distress or discomfort.

Survivorship: A Mixed Blessing

If taking medication for your mood feels very uncomfortable or wrong to you, of course you may refuse it; that is your right as a medical consumer. The decision is up to you, and only you. But many survivors feel that since they have already been through so much, and because they have more struggles ahead, anything that helps is welcome. As Phyllis, a member of one of our women's groups, said about her choice to take antidepressant medication, "I don't see it as a crutch, but, if it is, maybe I need a crutch until I can walk and run on my own again."

13. I received a flyer from my hospital saying that they're offering a support group for people finishing treatment. I'd like to go, but wonder whether it's only for people who don't know how to cope on their own?

It's tempting to respond to your question by saying "yes." But that's because cancer and its aftermath are a lot to cope with; there are very few people who could weather such an experience without the help of others. Many survivors tell us that they gain something especially valuable from talking to others who have been down a similar road. Although friends, family, and professionals may be supportive, they can't offer the same understanding and insight as can other survivors. A lot of people have gone through treatment feeling that they are the only ones to face the challenges of nausea and fatigue, the frustration of spending hours in a doctor's waiting room, or the pain of friends who are fearful or distant. When they become part of a group, they meet others who can understand and identify, because they've "been there." Suddenly, the world of cancer doesn't seem as lonely. Time and again we hear group members say, "No one understands like you guys." Even as seasoned professionals, we know we cannot offer the same kind of help.

It's important to note the difference between **support groups** and other types, such as **psychotherapy groups**. A support

Support group

A meeting, which may or may not be led by a professional facilitator, which brings together people with similar struggles to share their experiences.

Psychotherapy group

A form of therapy in which patients are treated for emotional problems in a group led by a mental health professional.

group will give you an opportunity to discuss your concerns and learn from others (including the group facilitators); it is not about changing your personality or receiving criticism from other members.

As you can see, we are great believers in the value of support groups for people who've been through cancer. Every time we convene a new group, we see all the special moments that occur as participants nod in agreement with one another or hand a box of tissues down to a tearful member. They are supplying to each other something that they could get nowhere else.

If there is a group for survivors available in your area, you might want to consider trying it out. There are also many online and telephone groups available. For more information, see the resources section at the back of the book.

14. *Is there anyone who* shouldn't *be in a support group?*

Yes. If you find it too painful to hear other peoples' stories about cancer and treatment, then you won't feel comfortable in a group. Some people tell us that they are quite impressionable, and that hearing about anyone's symptoms or fears will lead to them having the same ones. For them, groups are places to become more, rather than less, anxious and worried. Another person who might not choose a group is one who feels very responsible for the people around him. While a good group leader can help such a person not to work too hard caring for others in the group, it is sometimes simply too much of a challenge for the inveterate caretaker.

And, of course, your needs and feelings as a survivor may change over time; it may be that a group isn't the right thing for you at one point, but that it feels like a good option later on. Perhaps it could be helpful to speak with a counselor for a while on your own, and then determine, along with him or her, whether a group is right for you.

But again, although groups are not for everyone, they are helpful for the vast majority of people who have been struggling through tough times while feeling as though they are the only ones.

15. I find that ever since my treatment ended, I seem to have a short fuse. I'm snapping at my family, and I even got into a fight with a stranger in the supermarket. In fact, I almost feel like I'm looking for a fight! What's wrong with me?

Many people report the feeling you describe. Sometimes this reaction surprises them, because they think they should only have positive emotions about the end of treatment. But it is not really so hard to understand why there might be other feelings in the picture.

A patient going through cancer treatment has to be a "good soldier," marching through the rigors of chemotherapy or radiation with little chance to rest or complain. During this process, negative feelings may be set aside. It's only natural that such feelings might pop up after treatment ends, like a beach ball that has been held underwater for a long time. Sometimes this happens with a vengeance, surprising even the survivor and alarming those around him or her.

Somewhat connected to this phenomenon is that of clinical depression, which we've discussed previously here. Depression is often our response to loss, and the losses that accompany a cancer experience are many. Most people who go through illness suffer from the loss of their feelings of safety in the world. They may lose their sense of vitality and well-being. Many people treated for cancer undergo functional changes—some of these profoundly life-altering, like losing a limb. We have heard too, of how relationships may change or end. All of these factors (and more) can lead to a period of clinical depression, of which there are many symptoms. One might feel sad, crying often or in an uncontrolled way. One might have trouble sleeping or may sleep too much. Another symptom of depression can be marked irritability. You should certainly check this out with your doctor.

Finally, there is another condition connected to depression, but not identical to it, that may be involved. That is **Post-Traumatic Stress Disorder (PTSD).** In a sense, the term "disorder" is a misnomer, because it is only human and natural to have lingering distress after a traumatic event. But some survivors tell us that having a "diagnosis," for their feelings is actually helpful. PTSD is something that is often experienced by people who have gone through combat, a bad accident, or are victims of a crime. It can also apply to those who have been through a life-threatening illness and the grueling treatment that comes with it.

Post-Traumatic Stress Disorder (PTSD)

Psychiatric term describing the psychological aftereffects of very stressful or frightening events. Its symptoms may include irritability, memory loss, insomnia, anxiety, or depression.

16. One of my friends was recently was diagnosed with a recurrence of her cancer. I want to be a good friend, but I get anxious when I talk with her, and I find myself avoiding calling or visiting. Should I make myself reach out?

It's understandable that this situation poses a dilemma for you. Going to hospitals or discussing illness has a special meaning for people who have faced serious illness themselves. It is especially hard for cancer survivors to learn that someone's cancer has returned, because this is a worry that they must live with all the time. Spending time with someone who is sick again can heighten a survivor's worries about his or her own health, and may raise his or her anxiety to an almost unbearable level. You ask if you should "make yourself" reach out. Only you can answer this, since you know what will leave you feeling that you've been a good friend. But we hope that you won't be too hard on yourself if you choose to give

Some survivors have a post-traumatic stress response, like a soldier who has been through combat.

your support in ways that don't create too much discomfort for you. If calling is easier than visiting, do that. If you feel that you can't discuss your friend's illness right now, but want her to know you care, then you can send flowers, a gift, or a card telling her you're thinking of her. You may even want to go a step further, and tell her in a card or letter that you are having a particularly hard time hearing about her recurrence because you, too, are living with that possibility. Chances are, she will understand.

Judy, a 58-year-old survivor of lung cancer, comments:

I think that dealing with the worsening cancer of a fellow survivor is one of the most difficult issues there is. It's happened several times with me: each time in a different way, and each time I had a different response. The main question is how to be connected and caring without jeopardizing your own equanimity. Because although it is really just magical thinking, seeing someone else's cancer get worse is scary as hell— it's as if you could catch it, though you know better. You think about what it would be like for you: how it would feel, how it would look. So your compassion can get contaminated by your anxiety. For me, the hardest time was when a member of my support group became much more ill. I had always been concerned about her isolation, and called her regularly and accompanied her several times for second opinions. But when she became more and more ill, I began to feel overwhelmed by her despair: calling became very hard, and I would feel guilty for calling less. In a different situation, a colleague was diagnosed with lung cancer a year before me, and we shared the same doctor. My colleague died a year after I was diagnosed, and although it was hard to visit her as she was clearly becoming more ill, I was upset but less overwhelmed. I think this was because she was very closely connected to her family and friends. She was dying, but she was not despairing. So I guess I have learned that for me the idea of becoming more ill has to do with the fear of despair and isolation.

As ill people, we can try to stay connected to others and try to cultivate a community of family and friends to help each other help us.

17. My treatment wasn't too rough, and my doctor says it worked. I have a lot of energy and feel like I've put cancer behind me. My wife says I'm in denial. Is she right?

Your wife probably means well and wants to make sure that you acknowledge your cancer experience, rather than trying to sweep it under the rug. This is why she's raising the question of your being in **denial.** But you can reassure her (and yourself) that this isn't the case. The fact that you mention your doctor and your treatment tells us that you've attended to your health; those who are truly in denial simply hope their cancer will disappear, and this is not what you did.

We all live in denial to a certain extent. If we didn't, it would be hard to get through the day. Do any of us want to think that we might meet with an accident, be the victim of a crime, or lose a loved one? No—and yet all these possibilities exist. We "deny" them so that we can attend to the business of living.

You have said that you're feeling well, and that your doctor confirms that you are. This is great news. You sound ready to move on and enjoy life—go for it.

Denial

An emotional state that permits a person to keep painful facts out of consciousness in order to avoid the pain of acknowledging them.

PART TWO

Managing Uncertainty

Ever since my cancer, I feel so vulnerable. I feel like such a coward. Will I ever stop being scared?

Every time I have an ache or pain, I think the cancer is back. Will I ever get over that?

Why don't I feel happy when the doctor says everything is all right?

More . . .

18. Ever since my cancer, I feel so vulnerable. I keep thinking, "If cancer could happen to me, then anything could happen." Sometimes I'm almost scared to cross a street or be out after dark. I feel like such a coward. Will I ever stop being scared?

Feelings of vulnerability are common after cancer.

No one who has been through treatment for cancer should call herself a coward! However, the feelings of vulnerability you describe are very common after any type of trauma. One young woman said, "I feel like if I could get cancer, then one day a building could just fall on my head!"

You may have heard the expression Post-Traumatic Stress Disorder (PTSD). It is often used in connection with soldiers who have returned from combat or with someone who has been in a bad accident or witnessed a crime. These experiences remind people that, as human beings we *are* vulnerable, and can lead to the kind of generalized fear and anxiety you describe. In a simplistic version, this is a case of "once burned, twice shy." It is not unusual for the experience of a life-threatening illness, as well as very challenging treatments, to lead to a PTSD reaction. In fact, we see this fairly often—many survivors tell us that they feel nauseated when they even see an advertisement for their hospital or receive a piece of mail with the hospital logo, because they are reminded of their chemotherapy. Others say they can't bear to watch a television program or movie where cancer is featured. These anxious feelings may also generalize to areas unconnected with cancer. One woman developed a sudden fear of flying after her treatment; others are more afraid of traveling at night or being alone in the house. Over time, such feelings often fade. But if this doesn't happen, and you continue to feel so anxious, it could help to speak with a counselor who is familiar with cancer survivorship and who can help you put your experience into perspective. There are also a number of medications that are particularly effective for those who have PTSD.

Brian, a 31-year-old survivor of **sarcoma** comments:

My treatments left me feeling so weak and vulnerable that I had a huge amount of fear about my day-to-day activities. After surviving a most assiduous assault on my body, I had become terrified of dying from a simple fall down the stairs. Slipping in the shower, burning myself on the stove, or breaking a glass on the kitchen floor all seemed like they could have unimaginable consequences. (To say nothing of getting hit by the proverbial bus.) My confidence in my physical abilities was shattered.

But I'm slowly relearning how to walk and climb stairs; and I'm gaining the strength to open bottles and transport heavy boxes. I'm learning to operate in a familiar world in new and unfamiliar ways. As I accumulate these new experiences of self reliance, I am gaining confidence and letting go of some of the fear. The fear isn't fading quickly, but it is fading.

19. Every time I have an ache or pain, I think the cancer is back. Will I ever get over that?

In virtually every survivor support group we've had, someone raises this question. And in every group, heads begin to nod.

After someone has experienced a traumatic event—and a cancer diagnosis certainly falls into this category—it is natural that he become hyper-vigilant about his safety and well-being. If someone has been mugged on the street, he will look over his shoulder for a long time afterward. If someone is in a serious traffic accident, she may come to see cars as dangerous. This kind of anxiety is exacerbated in the case of a life-threatening illness, because it is our own bodies that caused us harm. Such fears naturally lead to a tendency to note every sensation and to worry that it is a harbinger

Sarcoma

A general class of uncommon cancers affecting the connective tissue of the body.

Managing Uncertainty

of illness. Survivors are hesitant to give up this process of monitoring their bodies. As one group member said, "Cancer snuck up on me. I don't want to be caught napping again."

Most survivors find, however, that over time, these anxious feelings recede. Slowly, they begin to trust their bodies again. For some people, the knowledge that they are being watched closely by their medical team is reassuring. This, after all, was seldom the case when the cancer originally occurred. Still others echo Lily, a 56-year-old colon cancer survivor: "What will be, will be. I want to enjoy the time I have with friends and family. None of us know what the future will bring."

20. I recently had a follow up–appointment and learned that everything was totally clear. Since the news was all good, why do I feel kind of down? And by the way, I noticed that this happened after my last clean bill of health too. Why don't I feel happy when the doctor says everything is all right?

Your question reminds us of a young man who was a "graduate" of one of our young adult groups. Whenever he had a follow-up appointment with his doctor, he would drop by to visit. One day he arrived, and when we asked how his appointment was, he sank into a chair and sighed "Well, I have six months to live." This answer didn't sound quite right, because we had no reason to believe Alex was ill and because few doctors make such predictions. When he was questioned further, he replied that this is how it felt to him—as if he were living from checkup to checkup. He felt that he could breathe easier for several months, but that as the next check-up neared he would begin to feel anxious and frightened once again. This feeling of being free only until your next appointment with the doctor may be part of what is getting you down. Perhaps it would be helpful to acknowledge that checkups and scans will be challenging, and to make a plan ahead of time to "de-stress" afterward—see a silly movie or have dinner with a good friend.

There can also be a let-down after any type of intense feeling. You may recall that the end of treatment itself wasn't the happy (or at least not all happy) occasion you thought it might be, either. It can take a while for your system to reset from a state of being on constant alert to a time of less urgency.

Give it a little time, and you may be able to integrate the fact that you remain well—and perhaps even celebrate a little.

21. I seem to spend all my time wondering what caused my cancer. My doctor and nurse say not to worry about that, but isn't it important to know so that I can avoid getting it again?

When something goes seriously wrong in our bodies, it is the most natural thing in the world to wonder how and why it happened. As you say, this is more than mere curiosity—it comes from a desire to avoid problems in the future. Virtually every survivor wants to know if there is something he should or could do differently in order not to be ill again.

In the case of some cancers, there are concrete answers to this. For those with lung cancer, or cancer of the head and neck, or bladder cancer, it is especially important not to smoke. This is because smoking can be a major contributor to these cancers. Even if your health care team does not believe that smoking contributed to your particular cancer, it is a good general health practice to refrain from tobacco use of any kind.

There are other substances used in industry and manufacturing that may contribute to some cancers. Other cancers have a strong genetic component. But that being said, the wisdom about what causes cancer and how to avoid it changes almost day to day, as we learn more and discard old theories. Hormones, coffee, and vitamins are three examples of things that have been thought to be helpful at some times, and useless or hurtful at others.

Many general guidelines about good health practices apply most especially to cancer patients and survivors. There is increasing evidence, for example, that exercise may be protective against breast cancer. And certainly, maintaining one's ideal weight and exercising can only be good for you. But if your health care team is not aware of the contributing factors in your particular case, it is probably best to stay as generally healthy as you can, and enjoy each day, without focusing on what are, for the moment, imponderables.

22. I'm a bottom-line kind of guy, so I asked my doctor point-blank what the survival statistics are for my kind of cancer. I was stunned when she told me that most people with my type of cancer get recurrences, and that most die of the illness! How do I live knowing that my chance of surviving is so poor?

It's easy to understand why you were so upset by what your doctor said. We turn to our doctors for hope and encouragement, but in this case you heard frightening news instead. The positive part of this is that you know your doctor will be honest with you and will tell you the truth to the best of her ability. But "the best of her ability" is the key phrase here. Most doctors will admit that they don't have a crystal ball and can't predict how any one patient will do. No one is a statistic, and that includes you. Even when two patients supposedly have the same diagnosis, they can't actually have the same disease. They begin with different bodies, respond

No one is a statistic, including you; even your doctor cannot predict how you will do.

differently to chemotherapy, and may even have a cancer that looks somewhat different under the microscope than someone else with the "same" disease. It is important to remember all this as you move forward. Another fact to bear in mind is that research is happening all the time. Medicines that are used routinely today did not exist when we began our career in this field. And while we are speaking of science, a final reminder: One well-known cancer doctor reminded us in a recent lecture that any statistic you read is already several years old. It is the result of studies begun years ago, and may be out of date by now.

The scientist Stephen Jay Gould, diagnosed with a very serious cancer called **mesothelioma**, lived for many years after his diagnosis, despite the fact that the statistics about his prognosis were not good. As a scientist, however, he was aware of how little the overall trend applied to any one person, and wrote at length about this. His own survivorship proved his point. And of course, many of us are familiar with Mark Twain's view that there are three kinds of lies: "Lies, damned lies, and statistics."

Mesothelioma
A rare form of cancer, usually caused by exposure to asbestos.

But there is another part to this answer: Part of being a cancer survivor is learning how to live with uncertainty. This seems like a daunting task when what you want most is reassurance and the sense that you are well, and will stay that way. But anyone who has received a diagnosis of cancer knows that there are no guarantees in life. Although in some ways this is a frightening experience, many survivors also say that it teaches them the valuable lesson of living in the moment. Those who have not experienced illness, pain, or loss may be less able to grasp the importance of this concept. But those who have been through the cancer experience are aware that in many ways, life is fragile and even fleeting for all of us. The most fulfilled survivors are those who learn to put this fact to use and to cherish small moments. A quick P. S. here—you can't do this every second of every day! Sometimes you will be mad that you missed the bus—or even deeply distressed about your health. But living in the moment is something for which we should *all* strive.

Brian comments:

This is essentially what my oncologist told me at the time of my diagnosis. It hit me like a ton of bricks, but instead of accepting it as a death sentence I challenged my doctor to suggest options. I asked him, "What can we do to make my outcome different?" Then I listened to his advice (and that of all my other doctors) and I listened to my body, and I have continued to make the choices that seem best for me given all available information.

I've pretty much given up trying to figure out how and when I'm going to die. I never really thought I'd make it this long. I was already dealing with two life-threatening illnesses before the cancer diagnosis. In reality, we all live with this terminal condition called mortality. It just seems like a waste of my time to stress about which disease will take me down for good. (For all I know it will be something entirely unexpected!) Instead, I try to focus my energy on how best to spend the time I have remaining here and now.

23. If my doctor says that I'm cancer-free, then why must I have such frequent follow-up appointments?

It's certainly understandable that you would want to put the painful experience of cancer behind you. Checkups can be a reminder that you were sick, and many people find themselves becoming increasingly anxious or upset as the date for their appointment nears. But maybe it would help to remember that seeing your doctor on a regular basis isn't about still being sick—it's a way of staying healthy. It would be irresponsible for your doctor to administer your cancer treatment and then say goodbye. She isn't seeing you because she expects you to become ill again, but rather to make sure that your treatment has done its job and that you are recovering well. It would be less than truthful to say that your doctor isn't also monitoring you for any recurrence of your disease; this is part of her job, and certainly part of the reason she will keep close tabs for a certain period of time. You may want to ask why certain tests or scans are necessary. It can be easier to go through such procedures when you know the rationale for them. If it's hard for you to ask such questions, or if you have trouble remembering the response, it may be helpful to have a family member or friend accompany you to your appointment. There are also professionals to assist you, such as patient navigators or social workers, who can help you strategize about learning what you want to know. After a while, your checkups will become less frequent—and it's even possible that you will miss them, as the next question indicates.

24. I actually want to see my doctor more often—better to be safe than sorry. But he doesn't want to see me for six months! Is that really OK?

Your doctor bases his timetable for follow-up visits on a number of factors. Usually, such a schedule grows out of scientific data relating to the type of cancer you had, as well as the type of tests needed to follow you. For example, your doctor may feel that it isn't possible to see the full effects of your treatment until a certain amount of time has passed. Or, there may be tests required to monitor your particular situation that are only helpful if administered at certain intervals. A **mammogram** given every month wouldn't be a helpful way to look at changes in the breast, for example (and would anyone really want one?).

It's understandable that you want to make sure that no symptom escapes your doctor's attention, and certainly if you feel that something isn't right, or if you have a question about your health, you should be in touch with his office to speak to him or a nurse. If you're finding that your doctor's recommendation is too hard to live with, then you could ask

Mammogram

A low-dose X-ray used to examine the breast, which aids in detecting disease.

Managing Uncertainty

whether more frequent visits are a possibility. If your doctor feels this isn't appropriate for you, then you might want to find a counselor who is familiar with cancer treatment and who understands how challenging it is to live with uncertainty. Together you might be able to develop some techniques to help you manage your anxiety.

25. I feel like I've adjusted to life after cancer pretty well. I'm back at work and enjoying time with my wife and kids. But every time I have a scan or test scheduled, my mood takes a dive. I have trouble sleeping and eating, and I feel edgy all the time. Does this mean I'm not coping as well as I thought?

The issue you've raised is such a common one that survivors have even invented a language of their own to give a name to what you describe. One of our women's groups included a French woman, Violette, who was very bright and intuitive. Though her English was limited, she always made herself understood and got the gist of what was being said by others. But one day Violette came across a word that stumped her. That word was "scanitis." "What is 'scanitis'?" she asked with a furrowed brow. The group laughed as various members began to answer her. They explained that it was a made-up word to describe the anxiety that survivors feel when facing medical tests. All members were in agreement that, even after they were months—or in some case years—after treatment, scans continued to be a challenge. A week or two before the scheduled date, they would notice a change in their mood. Some felt anxious, some depressed, some irritable and short-tempered. Upon reflection, many realized what was going on: scanitis.

Although it's never pleasant to feel anxious or upset, it can be helpful to realize that such a reaction to upcoming medical appointments is normal and *not* a sign that you aren't coping well. Once a test or scan has revealed cancer, it is understandable that one would be apprehensive about such events. Over time, you may come to expect this upswing in anxiety and be able to ride it out, knowing that it will pass.

26. Sometimes I think I'm doing great. I feel like, in some ways, I'm enjoying life more than ever after cancer. But every time I see a story about cancer or hear about a famous person who died of it, I feel horrible for days. Will it always be like this?

When you are in the process of recovering from cancer, it can indeed be hard to be reminded of any aspect of the illness. And certainly, one of the hardest things for any survivor is learning that someone has died of his disease.

Scans and checkups can be challenging; anxious feelings don't mean you aren't coping well.

When a friend or family member succumbs to cancer, it is inevitably painful and frightening. But many survivors tell us that it is harder when the person is well-known. "He had access to the best care, and he still died!" is often their reaction. When Jacqueline Onassis was unable to recover from lymphoma, many patients and survivors were deeply shaken. She was perceived as one of the most powerful and wealthy people in the world—and still she could not find treatment to cure her illness.

Sadly, cancer is a "democratic" disease, which can happen to anyone. This is one reason that your own friends and family may appear to be threatened by your illness. But it is equally important to remember that everyone's cancer is different. Even if someone has what sounds like the identical diagnosis, stage, and cell type, she is not you. Her genetics are different, the way her body responds (or fails to respond) to treatment is different. It can be frustrating not to find someone who is "exactly" like you—but it's also important to remember when you hear sad news that you are unique. If you are still troubled, it may help to discuss your concerns with a member of your medical team, who may be able to help you see that you are a "case of one."

27. I hate to bother my doctor. Is it okay to call him when I have a worrying symptom?

Therapist

A professional, often a social worker, psychologist, or psychiatrist, who assists people who are in emotional distress.

Hypochondriac

A person who worries excessively about being or becoming ill, often with no foundation.

A **therapist** who worked with cancer patients all his life said, "People who've been through cancer ought to be issued a license to be a **hypochondriac** that they can carry with them at all times. They should be allowed to just flash it when they enter their doctor's office." What he meant was that, once a person has been through a life-threatening illness, he should permit himself (and be permitted by his team) to seek reassurance or information whenever it is needed. As we've stated earlier, symptoms and sensations that might have been ignored in the past have a different meaning to someone who has had cancer. Remember, your doctor is your partner in managing your health after cancer. She can help you as you learn about new and different sensations, and can tell you whether a given symptom is something to be concerned about. Chances are that, after a while, you won't need as much reassurance. You will come to know your post-cancer body, and you will have a better sense of what to bring to your doctor's attention.

If feelings of worry and anxiety about your body don't subside over time, you might want to seek counseling with someone familiar with cancer. Working with someone in this way may help you to put your fears in perspective, and handle them in a way that takes less time and energy from your life.

Judy comments:

I feel fine about calling my doctor when I have any symptoms which trouble me, maybe in part because I don't have to call him—I can email him. I really appreciate the use of e-mail, because it saves us both a lot of frustrated waiting and calling time. If the problem requires a visit, he will tell me to set one up. But beyond the logistics, as a survivor with ongoing disease, I don't question the importance of calling attention to anything which concerns me. I would consider myself a bad collaborator in my treatment if I didn't.

PART THREE

Communicating with Family and Friends

I've been very hurt by an old friend's behavior. Ever since I got sick, she has completely disappeared. Should I tell her how hurt and disappointed I am?

Ever since my diagnosis, people I know ask me, "How *are* you?" with a sympathetic look on their faces. I'm getting really tired of all this sympathy! How should I respond?

Sometimes when I tell people that I had cancer, they ask things about my lifestyle before my diagnosis. I feel like they're blaming me for getting sick. Why do they do this?

More . . .

28. I've been very hurt by an old friend's behavior. Ever since I got sick, she has completely disappeared. She never calls, and she always seems too busy to talk when I call her. Should I tell her how hurt and disappointed I am?

The short answer is yes.

Many cancer survivors tell us that they have friends or family, formerly very close and caring, who just aren't there for them during their illness. The survivors' feelings about this may range from puzzled to angry—or beyond. And of course, it is puzzling, and even disorienting, to have someone you have always thought of as a fixture in your life be so absent just when you need them most. Some people even say "I found out who my *real* friends are!" This is an understandable reaction; we all want friends we can count on. If someone has hurt you terribly, only you can decide if you wish to keep that person in your life. But it's important to remember that all of us have limitations. A crisis like cancer reveals those limitations. Some people are terrified of hospitals or illness. Some of your friends or family may be so afraid of losing you that they "get lost" before this can happen. Again, you need to evaluate whether you can overlook or forgive their behavior while you are ill.

It's good, however, to see you use the words "hurt" and "disappointed." This is probably even truer than to say you were angry. Let your friend know how much you value her and how much you've missed her. If she's unable to respond to hearing that in a way that you're comfortable with, then you'll have to decide what place she has in your life. Perhaps she'll be a more casual friend. Perhaps you've found others you feel closer to. But the situation can't really be evaluated until you let her know how you feel.

Angela comments:

While some friends or family deal intuitively well with sickness, others need more direction. Many people really need to "do" rather than "be" when confronted with someone's illness. Friends like these often need specific things to do to feel helpful. That might be a chore or a task or a favor of some kind.

From my experience I found that it was important to determine realistically what people were capable of giving. Some are good at hand holding, others are good at distracting, others can whip up a great meal to deliver to your house. But there will be some that just cannot be there. Seeking out what people can give and letting go of unrealistic expectations helps lessen disappointments and can often renew relationships.

For those friends that are AWOL, their absence doesn't mean they have stopped caring or they don't want to know what's going on. Keeping them posted on how things are going, perhaps through someone else, can maintain that connection. And perhaps even improve the communication over time.

I lost some friends during my illnesses. I also regained some with time and work. But, for the most part, my experience has strengthened most of my personal relationships and made me a better, more empathic friend.

Reactions of friends and family may sometimes be hurtful; open communication can help heal wounds.

29. Ever since my diagnosis, people I know ask me, "How are you?" with a sympathetic look on their faces. I know they aren't asking an everyday question, but inquiring about my cancer. I'm getting really tired of all this sympathy! How should I respond?

Many cancer survivors tell us that they want very much for others to acknowledge their cancer experience—and to continue to acknowledge it, even after treatment ends. Others say they want to be "just like everybody else," and not looked on as a "cancer person." There is no one "right" way to respond to someone's cancer. Some survivors have even told us that they feel one way one day, and another way on another! One woman admitted, "Folks just can't win with me, let's face it!"

What we've found is that it is your reply to the type of question you describe that matters. If you're in the mood to forget about cancer and just be yourself, you can say "Great! How about you?" If you're in the mood for a little TLC, then you might say "Thanks so much for asking—I'm doing pretty well (or "not doing so well") today."

But, as we have said before, most inquiries from others contain at least a grain of genuine empathy, so, unless you think someone is truly insincere or sarcastic, a little patience may be in order.

Brian comments:

For me, the important delineation here is between concern and sympathy. I welcome the genuine love and concern that people feel a need to express now more than ever. But the pity and sympathy sometimes make me feel annoyed and resentful. It's usually pretty easy for me to tell from the tone of the question whether it's coming from a place of concern or pity.

If it's a concerned inquiry, I try to answer in a way that is appreciative and forthright about what I'm really going through at that moment. On the other hand, if I feel the question is being asked out of pity, I'll avoid the cancer issue altogether in my answer. Instead, I'll respond that "I just had the most wonderful massage," or "I have this annoying blister on my foot that's driving me crazy." This steers the conversation in a different direction; I find the look of pity disappears pretty quickly when I move into banal topics in this way.

30. Sometimes when I tell people that I had cancer, they ask things about my lifestyle before my diagnosis—did I have a lot of stress? Did I eat meat? Did I exercise? I feel like they're blaming me for getting sick. Why do they do this?

No one knows better than you do what a frightening disease cancer is. When you received your diagnosis, it may have hit home for the people around you; their own fears may have intensified. It may feel even more important to them to find out what substances to avoid, or how to behave in order to avoid getting sick themselves. This fearfulness is where their questions come from. After all, if they can find something that you do, or have done, that isn't part of their lives, they can tell themselves that they won't get sick the way you did. You know that isn't true, and maybe on some level they do, too. And it's easy to see how their questions may sound like they are blaming you—and perhaps they are, to a degree. But this is only because they want reassurance.

That being said, it is, of course, not your job to offer justification for your lifestyle or reassurance to others—especially false reassurance. No one can say with certainty what causes any individual case of cancer. Some lifestyle changes may reduce our risk, but no one is immune to cancer. When you are asked questions about your own lifestyle, you can either say you don't want to discuss this—or tell the other person that no one knows how or why you got sick and that cancer is something that can happen to all of us.

Susanne, a 29-year-old survivor of colorectal cancer, comments:

Being a cancer survivor makes you a lightning rod for other people's fears about their own health, and ultimately, their mortality. It becomes your fate to go around reminding people that they're going to die, and that they can't do anything about it. Quite a burden to bear! You try to live your life like anyone else, but again and again, against your will, you're the leper at the wedding.

For me, being diagnosed with cancer forced me to accept the randomness of things. I was in excellent health. I exercised, ate organic vegetables, and took my vitamins religiously. There was no family history. I was 28 years old! It made no sense. Early on, I asked my internist, a wise and wry doctor with decades of experience, why he thought this had happened to me. He looked me in the eye, and with great kindness said, "If I could tell you that, I'd win the Nobel Prize."

The laymen of the world are not so humble. They seem to think they might be able to get to the bottom of it.

I was at a bar for happy hour with a friend, and the bartender, a pretty girl around my age, overheard us talking about my hospital stay. She was interested. Which hospital, she wanted to know.

I told her it'd been to a cancer center.

"You had cancer?" she said.

"Yes. But I'm going to be okay."

"Do they know why you got it?"

"No. They have no idea."

"Well you should be grateful!" she said stridently.

My friend was disgusted that someone could be so insensitive. After all, shouldn't she be grateful that she doesn't have cancer? But I could see the terror in her eyes.

"I am grateful," I said. "Sure."

People are so afraid. They don't want to face what is obvious to us: to be alive is to be at risk for cancer, and all manner of mishaps and tragedies. We can only do so much to protect ourselves. Realizing that is actually a relief: instead of using up all of our energy trying to head off death, we can focus on being alive. If I'm grateful for anything, it's that.

31. I worry a lot about my cancer coming back, and I understand that's pretty normal. But whenever I express this to my husband, he says "Relax—you'll be fine!" This annoys me, because he doesn't know this for sure. Why does he keep repeating it?

In a sense, your husband isn't speaking to you. He's speaking to himself. It's likely that his constant reassurance is his way of telling himself that you will remain well. Your illness was probably frightening to him. He may even have thought he was going to lose you. These thoughts were so painful that he doesn't want to entertain them anymore.

It's hard for survivors to accept that the people closest to them can't appreciate and understand their anxieties. But these are often the *last* people who can listen to your health worries! This is a common stumbling block in survivors' most intimate and important relationships after cancer treatment. It's easy to get the feeling that those around you don't understand—or to be annoyed when they offer blanket reassurances that are not based in any knowledge, as your husband does. But it's also important to remember that your cancer affected those who love you, too. It's so easy to be caught up in one's own fear that those of family and friends get lost in the shuffle. Relationships *always* go more smoothly when you're able to see it from the other person's perspective; it's no different after cancer. So even as you tell your husband that what he's saying is not helpful to you, try to remember that he's worried too.

32. My wife has been a trooper since my diagnosis. She came with me to every doctor's appointment and every treatment, and has been so great that I hate to criticize her. It's just that every time I say anything about my cancer experience, she says, "I know exactly how you feel." How can I let her know that without going through cancer, she can't know how I feel?

It's clear that your wife has really been there throughout your treatment, and that the two of you have stayed connected. Her statement that she knows how you feel probably also stems from her wish to be connected. After all, the two of you are a couple, and until your illness you shared life as partners. Now you've had an experience that she really couldn't share. It's not that she couldn't help in some ways, or be by your side when the going got rough. But, as you know so well, it was you that had the cancer, you that took the treatment, and you that is the survivor. A survivor named Elizabeth said, "I really felt like I had great support leading up to my surgery. A lot of friends and family were even there on the day. But when they put me on the gurney and wheeled me to the O.R., I realized that I was the one who was going to go through the operation—and no one else." This felt very lonely to Elizabeth, and your situation may have felt lonely for you at times. But it may feel lonely for your wife, too. It may be quite hard for her to see you go through something that she can't really be a part of. That includes your survivorship, which you must negotiate in your own time, and in your own way. She may be afraid that your cancer experience will drive you apart in some way, or get between you. This may be why she's acting as though the two of you are one person.

You can remind your wife gently that your cancer experience was your own, and that while you both might wish that she could know exactly how you feel, she cannot. You can tell her that there are times when she has had experiences—like those labor pains!—that you couldn't share. But you also might reassure her that, nonetheless, you need her as much as ever.

33. It seems like whenever I tell people that I've had cancer, they tell me about someone they know who died of it. Why do they do something so insensitive?

When others are insensitive, it is probably because of their own fears.

We know that there are multiple challenges that cancer patients must face, both during and after treatment. Perhaps one of the most burdensome of those challenges is dealing with the fears of others. It is likely that you remember feeling fearful about the word before your own diagnosis. Although this may have changed for you, it is still true that when people hear the word "cancer," their anxiety often overrides their judgment. Their minds turn to their most frightening images of what the word means—and they may open their mouths before thinking. This is unfortunate, and, yes, insensitive.

The first thing for you to remember is that the person they are talking about has nothing to do with you. Even if that person had a similar diagnosis, she is not you. In many cases, she may have had her cancer many years ago, when treatments were very different. You may want to remind yourself of these facts in your own mind. Outwardly, you may choose to say, "I'm sorry to hear that your aunt didn't make it. But it's not helpful to me to hear that." You might want to add, "If you have any stories about people who are doing well, I'd love to know about them."

One survivor we know put a sign up on her cubicle that read, "If you have a scary cancer story, please don't stop by. Thank you. Cindy."

Having cancer may prompt you to reorder your priorities, placing more emphasis on what is most meaningful to you.

34. Since my treatment ended, I'm getting the same old requests to make something for the church bake sale, coach my kids' swim team, plan the office picnic, and carpool with other moms. I always used to say yes to everything. But now I just don't want to. Have I turned into a selfish person?

The powerful experience of having cancer often leads people to reassess their priorities, and reconsider what is important to them. For some people this means not reacting as much to the needs of others, and thinking more about what's meaningful to them. This is our birthright, and therefore is not selfish. Some cancer survivors even consider themselves fortunate to receive this reminder that we are allowed to make our own decisions about what works for us. But even if you're not feeling particularly fortunate at this moment, the fact remains that you owe it to yourself to really think about how you want to use your time and energy. Sometimes this is especially hard for women, who have traditionally been caretakers in the family and community. But men, too, tell us that they wish to set different boundaries. Both men and women say that they are not inclined to spend as much time at work, or to travel as much on business; these pursuits are not what matter most anymore.

One of our women's groups was struggling with the same question you raise—is it selfish to say no to requests and invitations? A group member suggested that a new word be coined: Self-FUL. Maybe that idea could be helpful to you. Kim, a member of a different group said, "Hey, if I have to, I'll even 'play the cancer card' to avoid something I really don't want to do! If I'm going to have this rotten disease, at least I should make it useful!" There may be times when you are truly too fatigued to participate in something, and you can mention this, if you're comfortable doing so. But these are techniques to use in the short run, while you continue to evaluate your priorities and decide what is meaningful to you. Over time you may get more comfortable saying "Yes" to what you want, and "No thanks" to what you don't.

Angela comments:

I found it took me a while to get involved again with day to day life. I was single and didn't need to work for a while so I had little pressure to get back to "normal" activities. Having had cancer gave me a mental permission slip for a small window of time. Permission to pursue things, do things, handle things on my own new terms. Life for a while had a tremendous clarity to it that helped me reorganize and prioritize things. It set a whole new course for me. And I cannot imagine how my life would have turned out without this gift.

Ironically, I knew that I was really getting better when that clarity began to fade. The small things started irritating me again. A whole day would go by when I didn't think about cancer. That sense of grand wisdom was not as consistently present. It was time to get on with a more ordinary, less glaringly lucid life. But that postcancer wisdom returns when life gets tricky and I need to make some serious choices.

So, what is the legacy of cancer as a survivor? Occasional bouts of intense fear, often followed by moments of profound clarity in the midst of a carefully crafted ordinary life.

Judy comments:

I feel I have a right and a responsibility to do as much as possible of what is joyful and fulfilling and as little as possible of what is cumbersome and burdensome. Which doesn't mean I don't have to do the dishes or pay my taxes, but it does mean that I can choose to say no to extra requests which I don't think will be good for me. Knowing I have a life-threatening illness has made me live more intensely and has made me choose more carefully to do what really matters to me. I have felt more excited about and more valuing of the things and people in my life which do matter, and I've been very open about communicating the enthusiasm and love I feel, which in turn has evoked a more open expression of love and generosity from others. Doing what matters doesn't mean being selfish, and it can sometimes mean being even more giving. It means being mindful about what you give, and deeply careful not to squander your energy and time—neither of which will last forever. For example, I turned down several offers to be on professional committees, since for me committee work is boring. But my husband and I have signed on to take care of the neighbors' 2-year-old boy, whom we love, when his mom goes into labor—which could be at any moment. That won't be easy, but I feel so lucky to have this gift of an intimate relationship with a 2-year-old.

35. My kids have always seen their dad as strong and capable. I just finished treatment and am pretty fatigued. My doctor says this will take time to get better, but isn't it important that I get back to normal quickly, so my kids won't worry?

It's very natural for you to want to protect your children and to give them all the time and energy you can. But when it comes to cancer, honesty is usually the best policy where kids are concerned. Children often tell us that they are aware of the gravity of a parent's illness, even when they haven't been told directly. This can sometimes make life frightening and confusing, because they may imagine things being worse than they are. They are likely to feel most reassured when people are straightforward about what's going on, rather than pretending that everything is fine, when they can see that this isn't the case. Let's face it, they know you pretty well, and probably know that you're not 100% right now. It's all right to tell them that you're on the mend and doing well—but that full recovery will take a while, and you're still tired. Depending on the age of your children, you can use different language. For a child younger than 7 or 8 years old, you might say, "The medicine that the doctor gave Daddy is really strong. That's good, because it helped me get better. But it's so strong that it also made me kind of tired, so I can't play as much as I'd like to right now." With an older child, you can be more straightforward, again stressing that you're on the mend, but that the powerful treatment you had has knocked you out, so tossing the football around will have to wait. One way you can remain the capable and in-charge guy that you've been is by proactively suggesting activities that you do feel up to—like watching a movie together, playing a board or video game, or reading to the younger ones. This way they'll know that you care, and that you want to be with them, even if strenuous activity is out for now.

36. My parents are in their 80s. I decided it would hurt them too much to learn I had cancer, so I never told them. Now my sister says I'm wrong to keep them in the dark. Who is right?

There is really no right or wrong answer here. First, you haven't said how well or impaired your parents are. If they have cognitive difficulties or are quite ill themselves, then it might be confusing or overwhelming for them to learn of your illness. Only you can judge that. And even if they are well and capable, your wish to spare them pain is understandable. Some survivors feel that for a parent to cope with a child's serious illness is a terrible experience at any age, and only harder for older people. Also, do they live at a distance? If this is the case, and there is little they could do to help—or to be reassured by seeing you well again—it is again understandable to decide not to share your illness.

On the other side, some people do decide that once treatment is over, they can say to elderly parents, "I went through a cancer experience, but it's over now. I didn't want to worry you, but wanted you to know now that I'm better." It could be, too, that you'll feel more like talking about your cancer once you have had time to adjust to the diagnosis, and integrate the treatment experience. People's reactions to their own disease are fluid, and may change over time.

Your sister genuinely feels your parents should be given the truth, and that they can handle this news. It might also be that she feels she is in an awkward position, knowing of your cancer, but having to keep it from your parents. So, if you continue to feel that you don't wish to share your cancer experience with your mother and father, you may want to acknowledge to your sister how tough it must be for her to be "in the middle," and tell her how much you appreciate her support here. This acknowledgment may be enough to help her support whatever position you choose. Remember, cancer affects not only the patient, but others in his life; they sometimes need acknowledgment, too.

37. My husband and kids were so supportive when I was sick. Now they expect me to pick up all the household chores, and chauffeur them everywhere again. I feel like they're so insensitive. Does this mean they don't care about me as much as I thought they did?

It must be confusing to get so much support during treatment, and so little once it ends. Since your family doesn't seem to be acknowledging all you have been through, it's understandable for you to conclude that they don't care about your feelings. But given what you say about their behavior during your treatment, it is unlikely that this is the case. More plausible is the possibility that they were all frightened by your diagnosis (as you were!), and worried when you were in active treatment. They are relieved to see you looking more like your old self. It may be that their renewed demands are their way of making sure you really are okay, and erasing the painful memories of your illness. One woman put it much as you did: "Before my illness, I would have told you I had the greatest kids in

Those who love and need you may pressure you to "get back to normal."

the world. But now that I'm post-treatment, they are brats! Leaving their laundry around, asking me to take them places. I guess I need to revise my opinion of the job I did with them!" After reflection, Amy realized that her kids weren't really brats at all, but were glad to see her treatment come to an end. Just like your family, they wanted reassurance that she was her old self. You know that this isn't possible; your cancer experience has changed you, in ways that may be painful, profound, or both. But this idea is understandably threatening to those around you. What they want most is the status quo. So, even though you know they can't have their wish, you may need to take a second look at their seemingly selfish behavior. And you may need to let them know, gently, that you want to help them and care for them—but the ways that you do that may not look just the way they used to.

38. My friends and family keep telling me how brave I was to go through such tough treatment. In a way this is nice to hear—but a part of me keeps thinking that they would have done the same thing if they had to. Are you really brave if you had no choice?

A lot of survivors tell us that the word "brave" doesn't sit well for them. Just like you, they say that they didn't choose to go through cancer, therefore, no matter what their response, it can't be called brave. One young man pointed out that a fireman who runs into a burning building is brave, because he deliberately chooses danger, whereas a cancer patient doesn't make that kind of choice. In some ways, that seems logical. But what if someone found himself in a bad train wreck or other disaster? Although one didn't choose this circumstance, one can choose the way that he responds. One can choose grace, dignity, even humor—as opposed to bitterness, anger, and self-pity. So, even though it may seem like you "had no choice," there probably *were* choices you made, which led people to admire you.

But it's possible that there is another level to your discomfort here. When people call you brave, it may feel to you as if they *are* implying you had a choice. This implication may tell you that they don't really understand or appreciate the way that cancer hit you out of the blue, giving you *no* choice in the matter. You may feel annoyed that they don't see that, in a sense, you were forced into your "bravery." This is understandable. For this reason, many survivors choose to say "You don't know what you might do in this circumstance," or "You would be brave, too, if you had no choice."

But remember, a compliment is a compliment, so you always have the option of saying "Thank you," as you recall all the challenging moments during treatment when you really did call on all your strength and resilience to get through.

Angela comments:

The question of bravery is very interesting. I was never comfortable with that description although it was often given to me. At the time I felt scared, overwhelmed, inspired, frozen with depression, manic with determination, raw with reality or numb with denial. But I never, ever felt brave.

Since then, however, I look back and realize that I was brave at times. I made brave choices and took chances that others might not have. I protected myself and took charge of my healing. I got on with my life and my plans in the midst of the chaotic interruptions of repeated illnesses. It's really only been with the passing of time that I have been able to own those accomplishments and embrace the bravery they required.

You may not have a choice in getting sick. But from then on, it really is about choices. We are all active participants in our treatments. This takes a large measure of bravery!

39. I find that ever since my cancer experience, I'm not as patient when friends talk about their problems. Sure it's tough to have a mean boss or to break up with a boyfriend. But try chemotherapy and radiation! What should I do when they want to share problems that seem trivial to me?

A lot of survivors talk about having the experience that you describe after their treatment for cancer. The problem they have faced has been so massive, the ordeal of treatment so overwhelming, that no daily problem can compare. A lot of them are tempted to say "Look—whatever's going on, it isn't cancer!" This is another example of how the experience of serious illness can shift a person's priorities, sometimes in ways that are confusing or upsetting to family and friends— and even to the survivor herself.

These feelings are understandable, and can actually be helpful in some ways. Linda, a woman in one of our women's groups, said that she used to spend hours on the phone with friends and relatives, patiently listening to their concerns and crises. After her cancer experience, she realized that her feelings had changed. Not only did some of her friends' concerns seem petty, but her time seemed more valuable as well. Linda told the group how much better she felt once she was able to tell her friends that she wasn't available to talk in the same way. In fact, the other members applauded when she said, "Now I realize that this is why God created phone machines!" Other survivors, too, celebrate the new perspective that cancer has given them about "not sweating the small stuff," and they tell us that this often extends to the problems of friends and family.

But, that said, most survivors do want to continue the relationships they have had prior to cancer. In order to do this, you do need to let friends know that their concerns still matter to you—even if those concerns seem petty or unimportant at times. Sometimes it's helpful to offer a disclaimer: "I'll try to help you decide which pair of shoes to buy. But I need to let you know that since my cancer, I know that this isn't a major problem. Let me lend you my new perspective!"

We all need the help of others at some point; no one can go it alone all the time.

40. I was so sick after my bone marrow transplant, I could hardly do a thing for myself. My friends, family, and neighbors ran errands, bought food, and accompanied me to the doctor. This was hard for me, because I hate being dependent on people! I feel like I need to repay everyone now, or else I'll feel like I took advantage. How can I do this?

It's clear that you value your independence and want very much to be able to function without the help of others. But the fact is, we are all *interdependent*. There comes a time in almost everybody's life when he or she needs help from others. This can be a challenging, and even humbling, experience—especially because we live in a society that values "toughing it out," and making it on your own. But asking for help from others is part of being human, and well worth doing. The good news here is that you have so many people in your life who care about you and want to be there in any way they can. Maybe it would be helpful to ask yourself if you would offer to help them if they had had cancer. And if you did, would you expect to be paid back? What you might want is acknowledgment of the help you gave; that is easy enough for you to convey to those who reached out to you.

It might be a real step forward for you to learn to accept the help you were given as something that people *wanted* to do.

Many people feel helpless, and even useless, when a friend or relative has cancer; they wonder what they can do to make a difference. When they find something to do, they often feel relieved. They may be glad that you let them help, rather than expecting something in return.

But if you feel that you must do something for your "team," you can do what one woman did and throw a party for those who were there for her. In her case, it included her nurses and her social worker. It happened that this woman loved to cook, but you don't have to take on such a big task—have it catered. And enjoy!

41. I have a 5-year-old daughter. When I needed surgery, I told her that Mommy had a boo-boo, and the doctor needed to fix it. She seemed to accept this, but I'm wondering—as she grows older, should I tell her what really happened?

It sounds like you've done a great job so far, giving your 5-year-old an explanation of your illness and treatment that she can understand. But, as Tara Leflein, LCSW of Memorial Sloan-Kettering Cancer's Kids' Express program says, you will want to revisit the issue, and more than once. She points out that as your child grows and develops, she will be able to accept a more complete and thorough explanation of what has happened. Leflein suggests that in a year or two you may be able to tell her that your "boo-boo" had a name, and tell her that it was cancer. You can tell her that cancer is something that doesn't belong in your body, and must be removed. Leflein suggests drawing a picture of your body, perhaps with the healthy parts in one color and the cancer in another. Explain that once it is gone, you are healthy again.

You might want to ask your child whether she has heard the word cancer. If not, you can explain, using the techniques

You will continue to discuss your cancer with your child as she grows, adjusting your language to her level of understanding.

we've mentioned. If she has, it is important that you ask her what she has heard, as some of what she knows may be scary or even distorted. If she says, "That's what Grandma died of," then you may want to stress that Grandma was older and sicker than Mommy, or that she had a different type of cancer.

Tara Leflein also notes that you must be particularly attentive to how a daughter responds to a mother's breast cancer. Some daughters become alarmed as they reach puberty, mistaking normal changes in the breast for indications of cancer. You can stress that it is normal for her breasts to change, grow, and perhaps even hurt at this time.

Finally, you will want your daughter to be aware of breast health and speak to her gynecologist about your health history as early as her teenage years.

But Leflein stresses that the most important thing you can do for your daughter is to let her know that you are open to her questions and concerns, and that she can come to you with any worries or confusion.

42. My friends were great when I was on treatment. But they're definitely not as understanding about after-effects. How can I get them to see that when I say I'm tired, it's not the same thing as when they say they're tired?

This may not be the response you wanted, but the answer is: You can't.

When we're feeling crummy, we really want others to understand. This is true, even on an everyday, non-cancer level ("If you knew what this headache was like, you'd see that I really can't get up and go today.") But the truth is that a sensation, whether physical or emotional, really can't be conveyed to another. Many survivors tell us that this is one reason that meeting others who have been through cancer is so meaningful; if you talk about fatigue with them, you don't *have* to explain. When you talk with friends and family, remember that not only is it hard for them to know how you feel, but they also have a strong wish for you to be well along on the road to recovery; this can lead them to downplay your discomfort or fatigue.

But the fact is, you don't have to explain to *anyone*. What you do need to do is to believe in yourself and in your right to stop when you're tired, opt out of an activity, or say no to an invitation. Sometimes the wish for others to understand is one way of getting "permission" from them to take a break. You don't need permission; or rather, you can give it to yourself. One of the useful lessons of cancer is that we must all treat ourselves as well as possible, and not wait for permission from others to do so.

Susanne comments:

When friends ask me how I've been feeling, they often seem to expect—or even want—a different answer than the one I usually supply. They are disappointed and alarmed and outraged when they hear that I'm still having a rough time.

"Does your doctor know about this?" they ask.

"But you're better than you were a month ago, right? You are getting better, aren't you?"

"This is ridiculous! You shouldn't still be feeling this way! Isn't there anything they can do for you?"

"Maybe you need to take vitamins." (Or keep a food journal. Go to yoga. Have biofeedback. And so on.)

Sometimes it's lonely. It sounds bizarre to say, but I almost miss my hospital stay and my long convalescence afterwards. My friends knew what to do when I was a wounded bird with an IV trolley, and when my days consisted of tiny bites of food, long naps, and slow creeps around the block. They could give me a foot massage, bring me magazines, or sit in bed with me watching DVDs. It was easy for us to feel close to one another.

Now my condition seems to cause them confusion and distress. I am in limbo: not sick, but not quite better either.

I know my friends are concerned because they care about me, but sometimes it seems like what everyone wants most from me is a neat and tidy story with a happy ending. I beat cancer! I am a survivor! I'm an inspiration to you all!

On one level, that's true. I fought—or actually, I think of it more as enduring—and I survived. But reality is messy. Real cancer stories are complicated, and they don't end when treatment does. I wish more people would understand that.

43. Whenever I tell people I had lung cancer, they ask if I smoked. As it happened, I didn't! I don't like their assumption, but feel like even if I had smoked, this would feel like blame. How should I handle this?

Many survivors of lung cancer face this question from others. And whether the survivor smoked or not, they don't appreciate it one bit. Those who were smokers feel blamed and may even have the sense that they are being told they got what they deserved. If they didn't smoke, they feel falsely accused and lumped in with those who did make a lifestyle choice that may have contributed to their illness. Again, when someone gets a diagnosis of cancer, those around him become alarmed. They want to be assured that this will not happen to them. Lung cancer is a disease that it is easy for people to reassure themselves about, because it is so closely associated with smoking. If someone doesn't smoke, they may feel immune from lung cancer. You know all too well that this isn't the case.

As with so many questions from others, you have choices here. You may feel so annoyed or angry that you choose to say, "I don't appreciate your question," or "Your question offends me." You might ask them how they would like it if they were sick and someone blamed them for it. Or, you may want to do a little education and tell them that you don't have to smoke to get lung cancer.

Judy comments:

I just don't get upset when people ask me if I smoked. In fact, I did smoke for about 10 years, but I'd quit for about 20 years before I was diagnosed. Although I feel sad that I smoked, I don't blame myself for having caused my cancer. Many times people who've asked the smoking question, acknowledge that they have been smokers and are worried about themselves. I tell them that many people with lung cancer either never smoked or were former smokers, and that the majority of people who did smoke never get lung cancer. Which is part of why I don't blame myself: I think that the main reason I got lung cancer was bad luck. I guess that if someone asked me about my smoking in a rude manner, I might say, "Why do you ask?" If they had a blaming attitude, I would say that even if a person was a longtime smoker until the moment of diagnosis, the person still did not "deserve" to get lung cancer.

44. My brother was recently diagnosed with an early cancer, which the doctors say is very easily cured. I'm glad and grateful for this—but I'm also kind of upset. All of a sudden I can't sleep, and find myself weepy from time to time. Why am I overreacting like this?

Don't expect that cancer will ever be a "neutral" topic for you.

For most people, cancer is not a neutral topic. But for those who have been there, it is virtually impossible not to have a strong and intense reaction to the subject. For this reason, the word "overreacting" may not apply to those who have been through their own treatment. There are many reasons for your emotional response to the news about your brother. Clearly you care for him and are worried, despite his excellent prognosis. As we've noted earlier, cancer can increase one's feeling of vulnerability, and may lead to a belief that danger lies around every corner. It may therefore be hard to believe that he will be all right. Your own health worries may also be increased by the fear that there is a genetic risk in your family, making it likely that you will get another cancer yourself. If this is the case, some clarification from your doctor may be helpful. You may even have the feeling that your own cancer experience started a sort of avalanche of bad luck for your family. Though this feeling isn't rational, it can be powerful, and may even include some sense of guilt for having "let cancer in the door." Finally, having cancer hit so close to you can bring back bad memories of your own treatment. You may feel that you're reliving your own experience of diagnosis and treatment.

This is a case where honesty is probably the best policy. You can let your brother know that, in addition to feeling bad for him, his diagnosis has made you anxious and upset. You can tell him to let you know how you can help, and also to tell you when and if he thinks your own bad memories may be keeping you from being helpful. Chances are he'll understand what you're saying—and may even express some of his own discomfort at making you go through this again.

45. I'm one year past my treatment for breast cancer. My sister recently had an abnormal mammogram—and I found out about this through a friend! It turns out that my family had decided not to tell me because they thought they needed to "protect" me. I was really angry at being left out and hurt that they thought I needed to be protected. You would think they would have wanted my input, because I know so much about doctors and treatments! How should I handle my disappointment in them?

As you know, cancer can be an isolating experience. It can leave you feeling that the rest of the world is standing firmly on the mainland while you drift on your own island, separate and alone. It's therefore understandable that now that your treatment is over, you very much want to be back in the world, a full participant in the life around you. This is especially true when your own family is involved. In this instance your family hasn't quite caught up to where you are. They obviously still have some anxiety about your well-being. Add to that their anxiety about your sister, and you have a group of very worried and concerned people.

While it must be hard to have your family continue to see you as sick or compromised, this may be more about them than about you. Your illness affected them too, and now they are further distressed by your sister's situation. Try to go easy on them, even as you let them know that you want to be included. Make it clear to them that you're eager to use the expertise you've gained from your own experience. This proactive stance will let them know that you are not a frail patient, but a knowledgeable and willing patient advocate.

46. I was found to have cancer when my son was just a year old. I was really wiped out when I went through treatment and had to rely on a lot of other people to look after him. Now he is really dependent on my husband. Did my cancer permanently damage my relationship with him?

Again, let's turn to Tara Leflein, LCSW, who helps many mothers cope with the effect that their disease has had on their children. She is not worried that you won't be able to have a full and loving relationship with your little boy. She points out that you can begin to reestablish an important connection with your son, even before you feel fully recovered. You can hold and cuddle him, put him to bed, or feed him, even if others are still providing a great deal of his care. As your energy returns and you resume your former activity level, you can become increasingly involved with him. You may want to avoid a common pitfall, and not attempt to reenter his daily world by being an authority figure. Let your husband be the rule-maker and disciplinarian for a while. You can be the source of good things like fun, food, and play. We imagine that your son is saying, "No" a lot these days— you don't have to!

And finally, remember that throughout family life there will be times when a child seeks out one parent more than another. When your son is 5 or so, he may be very eager to stay close to you, and at times may even say "Daddy go away!" to your husband. Even as this type of flux and change occurs, neither you nor your husband should fear that you are not both equally important to him.

PART FOUR

Legal, Financial, and Workplace Concerns

Do I have any legal protections as a cancer survivor?

I had to miss a lot of work when I was out on treatment, and I am about to return. Can my company fire me for being out sick?

I think I'm being discriminated against because of my cancer. Should I hire a lawyer?

More . . .

ADA (the Americans With Disabilities Act)

Legislation passed in 1991 to ensure that people with health problems—or a history of them—do not suffer discrimination in the workplace or elsewhere.

Essential Functions

Legal term referring to those aspects of a job that are integral to performance of the job.

Reasonable accommodation

Legal term referring to the special allowances, structures, or schedules that a workplace must make to a disabled worker.

Undue hardship

A legal term referring to loss or damage suffered by a person or company as a result of providing accommodations that they cannot afford.

It's important to learn your rights under the law as a cancer survivor.

47. Do I have any legal protections as a cancer survivor?

Cancer patients and survivors, as well as others with medical conditions, are protected under Title I of the **Americans With Disabilities Act (ADA),** which took effect in 1992. The act prohibits employers from discriminating against people with disabilities in the workplace. It includes the application and hiring processes, and well as cases of advancement, promotion, and pay raises. A person is protected under the ADA if he or she has a current medical condition, a history of one, or is *perceived* as having any type of medical impairment. This last provision may be especially applicable for cancer survivors, because a boss or supervisor who is uninformed about cancer may think that a survivor will not be strong or well enough to do a certain job merely because she has had cancer—or may believe that someone who has had cancer is sure to be sick again. The ADA protects you against these unwarranted suppositions.

The law assures that you cannot be discriminated against when you apply for a job or when you already have one. You are considered qualified for a job if you are able to perform the *essential functions* of that job, or if you can perform those functions with **reasonable accommodation.** Reasonable accommodation means that your employer must make an accommodation to your disability, as long as it does not impose an **undue hardship** on that employer—that is, as long as it doesn't require expense or effort that is not commensurate with the size and resources of the company. (For example, a small "mom and pop" store is not required to provide a specially equipped car to its delivery person. But an office in a large corporation can certainly furnish you with special seating, or a computer screen that is adapted for those with visual problems.)

48. I had to miss a lot of work when I was out on treatment, and I am about to return. Can my company fire me for being out sick?

In most cases, no. There are exceptions, however, which mainly have to do with questions of what is undue hardship. If, for example, a person is the head designer for a line of clothing and will be out for an indeterminate amount of time, then it wouldn't be easy for the company to find someone of their caliber to fill in temporarily. It would pose an undue hardship to the company not to have any new designs created while they were away. Similarly, if you were the star soprano for a small opera company and had to be out for a long period during the performance season, it might be too difficult for the company to find someone else who could perform key roles. There are other such examples, but, in the main you must be offered a *comparable* job to the one you had held. The law does not require that you be offered the *identical* job you had before your absence; a lateral move is acceptable. It must, however, be a position with equivalent pay, benefits, and responsibilities to the one you previously held.

49. When I was ready to return to work after treatment, my boss told me that there had been a restructuring of the company, and my position was eliminated. I don't believe that, and think I'm being discriminated against because of my cancer. Should I hire a lawyer?

That depends. If you are considering legal action, a few caveats are in order. The first is perhaps the most important: If you wish to make a case for discrimination, your superiors (or at least your supervisor) *must* be aware that you were treated for cancer. It is not possible to claim that your cancer history was used against you if no one in the workplace was aware of your medical situation—even if you think they may have heard about it through the grapevine. This cannot be stressed enough, and it does argue for sharing your need for treatment with your direct supervisor, even if you would rather keep it to yourself. This does, of course, carry some risk; we have admitted above that the information may be used to deny you advancement. But it becomes invaluable in making the case that discrimination was at play. A catch-22 in some ways, but one you should be aware of.

Second, it is very helpful for you to keep a record of episodes that you feel reflect prejudice or discrimination. Make a note of dates and of what occurred. This will be helpful in supporting your claim, whether the information is used by you, or, more formally by your attorney.

Finally, you must demonstrate that you were treated differently from others at the job without a history of cancer. If *everyone* was moved to offices without windows, or if there is a massive layoff including many others, it will not be easy to claim that you were singled out.

One survivor who called us for advice presented a situation that reflects several of the principles outlined here. She had been laid off in a massive cutback at her company. She went to her supervisor and said, "This is a special hardship for me, because I just finished treatment for cancer." She described her supervisor by saying, "Her jaw just dropped. She had no idea." The survivor was wondering whether she could make a legal case for prejudice. In her case, this was unlikely because 1) many "well" employees were let go at the same time, and 2) she had not informed her supervisor of her medical situation until after the layoffs were announced. It's clear to see that this was not a situation that lent itself to legal action claiming discrimination.

Incidentally, what this woman decided to do was to approach her employer and simply say, "This is a hardship for me, because of my recent bout with cancer. Could you delay my release date in order to extend my benefits?" Many survivors have found this course of action successful. Frankly, when employers are aware of someone's cancer history, they often choose *not* to include that person in cutbacks, as they don't wish to create even the appearance of prejudice or hard-heartedness. This is an instance where prejudice can work in favor of survivors (Though by no means is this always the case).

50. I'm interviewing for a new job. Do I need to tell prospective employers that I had cancer?

Many survivors are under the impression that they are required under the law to disclose a history of cancer. We cannot stress strongly enough that this is *not the case.* As we have mentioned previously, cancer patients and survivors are protected under the Americans With Disabilities Act (ADA), which assures that they cannot be asked about whether they have a disability. Unfortunately, many survivors feel that they are being less than honest if they don't mention their illness and treatment. For this reason, we suggest that you rehearse the interview process with a trusted friend. This will help you manage your urge to "confess" your cancer history—as well as helping you to decide how you *do* want to present yourself to someone for whom you'd like to work. Sometimes a survivor's anxiety about his cancer history prevents him from remembering the qualities that would make him a desirable employee. Take time to do that before your interview, and be sure to remember your rights under the law. The fact is your cancer history is your own business, and not the concern of someone who is thinking of hiring you. You should know, however, that a prospective employer can ask you about your ability to perform tasks that are an important part of the

You do not have to tell a prospective employer about your cancer history.

job—for instance, "Could you load heavy cartons on to a truck?"

When we discuss employment further, you will see that some people *choose* to mention their cancer experience, as they feel it has been an important part of their personal development. They may feel that all they have gone through only serves to make them a stronger and wiser person, and that this growth can only help in whatever job they are hired for. This level of openness is certainly an option—but it is not a requirement. It may be that so many survivors think they must mention their cancer because it *is* imperative that you share your history with a new insurance carrier. For more information, refer to the following question.

51. I know it's illegal for a prospective employer to ask about your health status, but what if they do so anyway? Wouldn't it seem defensive to say, "You can't ask me that?" How should I handle this?

As we've stressed previously, a prospective employer is not entitled to information about your health history and is not permitted under the law to inquire about it. But you are wise to be prepared for such a question, should they ask anyway.

The most important thing to remember is that, if you are applying for a job, this fact alone means that you are ready, willing, and able to work. This is something to bear in mind as you respond; it is your motivation and wish to work that are key. Knowing this, you can once again go one of two ways. You might choose to disclose fully, and say that you have recently had a bout with cancer, but have been cleared to work and are eager to get back. As previously mentioned, there are people who feel most comfortable taking this course of action—and some employers who will value such an approach. But you also have the right to simply answer the question with what is true *as of that moment.* If you are filling out a form with check boxes, you may check "Good" or "Excellent," depending on what appears. Remember that you are answering as of *that day*—not 3 months ago when you were in the middle of chemotherapy.

You may be aware that you're still experiencing some aftereffects of treatment (to be discussed in another section), and feeling that it is dishonest not to disclose these physical challenges. But again—remember there will be other job applicants who suffer from poor eyesight, weak ankles, hearing loss, or other symptoms that they don't feel they need to share in an interview situation. You have the same right to keep your own physical challenges to yourself.

Finally, we must stress again that when it comes to your health history, the place where you *must* disclose is when providing information to a new insurance carrier, after you are hired. Not to do so is to commit insurance fraud—and you don't need that!

52. What if I'm hired? Must I disclose my cancer history then?

No. There is no need for an employer to *ever* be informed of your cancer history. As we've stressed previously, the people who must be given full information about your health are those at your new *insurance company.* They are not permitted to share this information with your employer.

Some people do choose to share their situation with an immediate supervisor, in order to enlist his understanding of the need for follow-up care or checkups. These people prefer to tell the person they report to that they will require schedule flexibility in order to keep up with their medical care. They stress, however, that they wish to do this in a way that disrupts the office as little as possible. Taking such an active stance shows your supervisor that you are committed to your job and want to be a responsible employee. It is always good advice to go to your boss with a solution rather than a problem. Most supervisors will be impressed by the fact that you have given thought to the issue.

Also, if you should ever feel that you are being discriminated against in the workplace because you are a survivor, it is important to ensure that someone in administration is aware of your cancer history; such disclosure can protect you against unfair treatment.

53. Ever since I returned to work, I notice that people treat me differently—almost like they're afraid. The other day I saw someone wiping off my telephone before they used it! Do they think cancer is contagious?

Unfortunately, cancer is still so misunderstood that some people may actually believe it is contagious. Even if they know better, people faced with cancer may be so anxious about it that they become irrational. They may want to do *something* to insure they will remain healthy, and therefore treat cancer as if it is a cold that they can avoid with proper hygiene. The avoidant behavior you describe may indeed come from a belief that people can somehow protect themselves if they keep their distance. But this is a complex phenomenon. In one of our support groups, a woman described the kind of behavior you've noticed among her own friends, and wondered also, if they believed they could "catch" her disease. Paula, a wise and funny member of the group responded, "Well—my friends are too smart and sophisticated to think they can catch my illness—but some of them seem to think they can catch my bad luck!" She went on to say that her analysis was based on something she had noticed when a member of her crowd was widowed. Other women seemed to back away, afraid that somehow they, too, could meet her fate. "The attitude seemed to be 'If it happened to her, it can happen to me,'" said Paula. "I think this applies to cancer, too."

Several other survivors have wondered if people's distance comes out of a feeling that the survivor will not be around much longer, and that there is little point in connecting with someone who will soon disappear. This outdated view of cancer may stem from things perhaps learned in childhood at a time when cancer was a much less treatable illness than it is now. Some people may have seen too many "Movies of the Week" where, in order to provide a dramatic story, cancer equals death.

This explanation of people's standoffishness may not offer much comfort if you're feeling isolated and alone. But perhaps it can prevent you from being distant in return, and can permit you to do a little education, explaining that your illness was appropriately treated, you are now healthy, and that in any case, your doctor has assured you that you pose no risk to anyone else.

There is an addendum to our answer. Many survivors have told us, "I know that I have the ability to educate people about cancer—but with all that I have to handle, I don't feel like being a teacher, too!" This is understandable, and we want to stress that you don't *have* to take on this role. It is simply one way of handling the ignorance and fear of those around you.

54. But I'm not just worried about how I'm treated by coworkers; I also don't want people to think I'm not up to the job—or to deny me a promotion. Aren't those fears realistic?

Unfortunately, cancer survivors do often meet with this type of prejudice; this can't be denied. Having laws in place to protect you is a wonderful thing, but you can't legislate attitudes and beliefs. There are still many employers who believe that people who have been treated for cancer are not able to work at the same level as others, and, sadly, some who believe that a person who has had cancer will soon die of the disease. This can lead to subtle forms of prejudice, which are hard to battle. It is difficult to prove that you didn't get a promotion because you had cancer—but not impossible. One young man in a support group was specifically told, "We're going to give the promotion to someone else, since we want you to rest and recover this year." In his case, his employer made a statement which reflected that a) this young man's cancer history was part of the decision not to promote him, and b) that the supervisor didn't know the law! In this particular case, he decided to pursue legal action. (Although it should be noted that this decision was not made lightly. After going through the rigors of medical treatment, he wasn't sure he wanted to expend the time and energy needed to participate in preparing his case. He finally decided that it was something he needed to do, and even said, "In some ways, I feel that my full emotional recovery depends on it." This doesn't mean that this decision is right for everyone.)

You cannot be denied a promotion based on your history of cancer.

But once you become aware of the protections afforded you, it is unlikely that legal action will be required in order to handle workplace prejudice. Chances are, if you let your boss know that you are aware of the law, and educate yourself, you will not need to resort to a lawsuit.

55. I decided not to tell anyone at work that I had cancer, because I didn't want to be pitied and gossiped about. I think I did the right thing. Did I?

Each survivor has to decide for himself how open he wants to be about his cancer, and there is no right or wrong choice. Some people are deeply private, whereas others tend to share personal issues more freely. In one support group a woman said, "I choose not to share my cancer history with anyone." Another woman piped up, "Are you kidding? Yesterday I told everybody at the bus stop!" Very different choices!

Having said that there is no right or wrong way to handle the information about your cancer, let's look at some of the reasons you give. It's true that cancer is a subject that most people have a pretty strong reaction to. Though we all know that cancer is common, we all hope that it will not affect us or anyone we know. When it does, it can indeed be the subject of comment. But, in our experience, the reaction of most people is empathy and sorrow that you are ill, which are not the same as pity. The word "pity" implies that people are looking down on you in some way. Empathy means that people are putting themselves in your place and saying, "Wow, that must be rough." Sometimes, when we're going through a hard time, that kind of response can be meaningful and can help us to feel less alone. It goes without saying that the more people who know about your cancer situation, the more support you can call on. We have seen that survivors who do choose to share their cancer story, who have an "open door policy" at work, giving permission to others to speak about and ask about their cancer, often get an outpouring of support that those who are more private do not. But again, the choice is up to you.

56. I used to enjoy hanging around the water cooler at work talking about silly things like office gossip, the local sports teams, or popular TV shows. But now this seems meaningless and unimportant. How should I handle it when these conversations begin?

As we can see from questions like this one, many survivors find that the experience of cancer has changed them in deep ways. In addition to some of the anxious and sad feelings that may come with the experience, there can be a renewed sense of what matters in life. Many survivors describe this feeling as liberating and rewarding, allowing them to not sweat the small stuff, and to worry less. But it can also prove difficult when everyday conversation feels superficial or empty. After all, light conversation is a way that people connect to one another, especially in the workplace. It gives coworkers the opportunity to reach out to each other and form a community, without necessarily sharing their innermost thoughts. This community is a source of support and comfort that many of us find gratifying; light conversation is the "glue" that holds it together.

We're not suggesting that you spend hours of your time in discussions that hold no interest for you or that you behave in a phony, inauthentic way; however, if you distance yourself from those who chat about lightweight topics, you may find it harder to feel part of the workplace community, and you may feel isolated at a time when you need the company of others. Also, your coworkers may misunderstand your distance as disapproval. Although this may be the case, it is still not really in your interest to remove yourself totally from such group conversation. Can you find a middle road, perhaps not participating, while at the same time smiling at some of the foolishness that is discussed? Could you find one topic that does have meaning for you—like what a beautiful, crisp weekend it was, and how good it felt to be out in the sunshine?

It's true that some water cooler conversations really *aren't* very substantive. But such talk greases the wheels of our society. It may be worth it to give a try. When you really cannot do so, retreat unobtrusively to your workspace.

57. After my cancer diagnosis and treatment, I lost my job and now the bills are really piling up. How do I get help out of this major debt?

There is no question about it: Cancer can be an expensive disease. Even with fairly comprehensive health insurance coverage, you may be burdened with noncovered medical expenses, as well as things like additional child care, or transportation costs. If you're not working and are not covered by disability benefits (or even if you are), you can indeed get pretty far into a financial hole.

The first thing to remember, as with so many things, is not to panic. No one likes to get letters from a collection agency, and the last thing you need on top of the stress of illness, is bullying phone calls from creditors. But this is a time when you need to take a deep breath and strategize.

If your income is truly low or nonexistent and you have few assets, then be aware that you can apply for public assistance which will supply cash and food stamps. We realize that this isn't an attractive prospect for many people, especially if working and earning your way has been important to you. But don't forget that this is a safety net the government provides for times such as these; if you are eligible, then don't hesitate to take advantage of this benefit.

If your financial resources are not low enough to qualify you for public assistance, there are still things you can do to take off the pressure.

Remember that creditors would rather be paid something than nothing. Many patients have been successful in getting in touch with creditors and saying, "I am being treated for cancer" (or "have just been treated for cancer"). They may then ask for their total debt load to be reduced, or request that interest rates be lowered, or that the clock stop ticking on interest. Again, creditors respond to this, because they hold out hope that once the crisis is over, they will get something from you.

Some people borrow from family members and repay the debt once they are back on their feet. For many people in our "rugged individualist" society, it feels hard to do this. But remember—many of the people around you are wondering how they can help. Sometimes you can give them a very concrete way of doing so.

Don't let creditors panic you; take a deep breath and strategize.

58. Can I get life insurance now that my treatment is over and my doctor says I'm free of disease?

Getting life insurance after a cancer diagnosis is obviously going to be a different prospect from applying for it with no history of serious illness. Still, it isn't out of the question. Different insurance companies take varying approaches on this question, but in general, the answer depends on the type of cancer you've had, and on how long you have been cancer-free. Some carriers may say that you must have been out of treatment for at least 5 years. Others will be more specific about the type of cancer you have had, frankly looking at the rates of recurrence of that cancer. This can be especially annoying because no survivor wants to see himself, or his prognosis, as a statistic. But remember, we're talking about insurance companies! They base their entire industry on actuarial tables, and none of us is free from their speculation on our life span.

Sometimes people can get life insurance through their employer "no questions asked." But this is the exception, and you should be prepared to shop around in order to find the carrier willing to work with you.

59. Since finishing my treatment, I've decided to leave a job I never liked much in order to pursue a lifelong dream—in the fall I will start teaching school. But it's only April, and I'd like to leave my job now to rest and prepare mentally. My only worry is, I'll still need health insurance, and won't be on my new plan yet. What can I do?

In most cases, when you leave a job, you are entitled to continue your insurance coverage under a provision called **COBRA.** COBRA stands for the Consolidated Omnibus Reconciliation Act, which was passed by congress in 1986, in order to provide continuation of group health coverage beyond the point where it might ordinarily end.

This allows you to remain on your former employer's group insurance plan for 18 months. Please note: In order to benefit from COBRA, you must have been working for a company with 20 or more employees that has a group plan. Be aware, too, that once you exercise the COBRA option, *you are responsible for the cost of your insurance premiums.* The price is the cost to the company to insure you, plus a few percentage points more to cover administrative costs. It is not cheap, but well worth it to make sure you are continuously insured—and in most cases, cheaper than purchasing insurance outside a group plan. Be sure to discuss this with your Human Resources Department before you leave. (Note: In some cases, COBRA may be continued for 36 months, for example, if you have or adopt a child. Be sure to find out what these exceptions are.)

You may also qualify for state-specific government-subsidized programs, depending on your income.

Finally, in most states, you can purchase an individual policy. Shop around as the cost of premiums, as well as the extent of

COBRA (Consolidated Omnibus Budget Reconciliation Act)

Law passed by congress in 1986 providing continuation of group health coverage that might otherwise be terminated.

In most cases, you cannot be denied health insurance because you had cancer.

coverage may vary widely. And be aware of what is important to you. Is prescription coverage something that you want to be sure to get? What about coverage for psychotherapy? Again, you are as much of a consumer when shopping for insurance as for anything else. Do not think of yourself as having to settle for anything because you are "lucky" to get insurance.

60. Won't I be denied coverage, due to having a preexisting condition?

Be aware that, in most states, you can purchase an individual policy, which will cover **preexisting conditions**, provided that you have not had a lapse of more than a certain number of days. This number varies from state to state, so it is important that you learn the guidelines for yours by calling your state department of insurance. This time period will be important to you, because the last thing you need is to be without insurance. Remember that even though your cancer has been treated, you will need to be followed closely in order to stay healthy.

Preexisting conditions

Term used in the insurance industry to describe medical conditions that existed prior to your being covered by a particular carrier.

The question of having continuous coverage with a gap no longer than that allowed by your state is important even if you obtain a policy via a new employer. Preexisting conditions may not be excluded from coverage, *as long as you have not let your insurance lapse* for more than the allotted time period for your state.

61. I'm a really efficient executive secretary at a large insurance firm; I type 120 words per minute, set up a new filing system that saves my boss a lot of time, and keep his schedule. But one of my tasks has always been to move heavy boxes of copier paper. Now my doctor has told me that, because of lymphedema in my right arm, I should not do this anymore. Can my boss still make me do it?

No. The key phrase here is "reasonable accommodations." It is incumbent upon your employer to offer you help with tasks that your disability prevents you from doing, as long as you perform the essential functions of the job. It does not sound like moving heavy boxes is an essential function here. The main component of your job is using your considerable business skills. It sounds like a reasonable accommodation for you would be for your boss to reassign the moving of the copier paper to someone else in the office, who does not have your physical limitation. Or alternatively, to provide you with a cart or other conveyance that makes this task easier to perform.

It's important to note that you mentioned working at a large company. If you had said that you worked in a small business, perhaps made up of your boss and yourself, he might *choose* to provide you with help—but he would not be *required* to under the law, if it represented a hardship to hire another person or purchase new equipment. (Let's hope he would offer to pitch in and move it himself!)

62. The other day my boss told me he was taking me off a project that I've been working on all year. He told me that he didn't want me to be under too much stress and was worried that the late nights might be too much for me. Is this discrimination?

Maybe yes, and maybe no. The answer depends on a few variables.

Did your boss state that his concern was based on your cancer history? When he used the term "too much for you," did you ask what he meant? Even if you feel fairly sure that he was alluding to your illness, that isn't enough to actually prove you were discriminated against. Another key question is, of course, did you inform your boss that you had cancer? If not, even if you think he "heard it through the grapevine," it would be difficult to prove that he knew, and was basing his actions on this knowledge. This may be true even if you informed your immediate supervisor of your history, and feel sure that he shared the information. Again, this cannot be proven.

But if you notice a *pattern* of behavior, where your boss is consistently removing you from projects, excluding you, or bypassing you, be sure to *keep notes*, with dates and examples. You may want to have a special notebook just for this purpose. Then consult an attorney who specializes in employment discrimination, and see what he or she has to say.

Sometimes honesty is the best policy when there's a gap in your resume.

63. I was out of work for a while, getting treatment for my cancer and then recovering. Now there's a gap in my resume. How do I explain this to a prospective employer?

This is one of the most commonly-asked questions in our survivor meetings. Although some people are able to work throughout their treatment, or at least remain employed on paper, others must take considerable time off, which is then reflected on their resumes. There's no question that such a gap does present problems. We know that there are some prospective employers who will automatically dismiss a candidate whose resume has time unaccounted for. But recently, when we invited members of a major financial institution to speak to survivors about their resumes, we learned some surprising things. Although most of the panelists said that they would be very concerned about a gap, they also said they would respond positively to someone who was honest about the reason they were not working for a period of time. They added that they would be impressed both by the person's honesty, and by their getting through a challenging experience like treatment for cancer. Of course, this is not a guarantee that being upfront will get you a job, but it's something to consider. In fact, one survivor we know turned his cancer history into a positive during his interview. He said, "If I can get through a bone marrow transplant, I can do anything this job asks of me!"

Some survivors find ways to fill the gap. But before discussing those, we must emphasize that you should *never* lie on a resume. If such a lie is discovered at any point, it may be grounds for dismissal. And besides, do you want to have to maintain a lie? You need all your energy to do your new job! That being said, we have known survivors who have truly plausible reasons for being out of work—such as staying home with a young child, or writing a book, and they include these explanations in their cover letter. But again, the reason must have a basis in truth.

Finally, we have one more suggestion. It's a good idea to remain connected to your field in some way, even when you're still not working. If you can, attend a conference, subscribe to a newsletter, or stay in touch with colleagues. This will show a prospective employer that your interest in working is sincere and that you care about keeping up with your profession.

But I just started my job a month before I was diagnosed. How long do you have to work somewhere before you are covered by the Americans with Disabilities Act (ADA)?

You are covered by the ADA no matter how brief the length of your employment, as long as your workplace has 15 or more employees.

I was fatigued when treatment was over, so I asked my employer if I could work from home. She said this would not work, because part of my job is meeting customers face-to-face. Doesn't she have to make an accommodation for me under the Americans With Disabilities Act?

No. Your boss seems to be saying that in-person meetings with customers are an "essential function" of your job. The ADA specifies that accommodations must be provided as long as you are performing the tasks central to your job. As much as you would like to work from home—and may even feel that it is possible to maintain your level of involvement with your work by doing so, your boss has the last word on this one.

64. I am still feeling tired and sick from the treatment and am finding it really difficult to function at work, can I apply for Social Security Disability (SSD)?

You can certainly try to obtain SSD, but it is unlikely that you will be successful based on your **post-treatment fatigue**. In general, the definition of disability according to Social Security is the inability to work for at least one year, which your doctor would have to attest to and explain—*or* having an illness likely to result in your death. Fortunately, most post-treatment after-effects do not fit in the latter category, and few in the former. In our experience, those cancer-free patients who apply for SSD during the post-treatment phase are rarely successful.

Post-treatment fatigue

Marked lack of energy or stamina following treatment for cancer; this may be radiation, chemotherapy, surgery, or any combination of those.

What you might be able to do is to obtain **Family and Medical Leave** for some period of time, if your doctor agrees that you need to rest. The **Family and Medical Leave Act (FMLA)** is a federal law that provides you the right to keep your job if you take time off to care for a sick family member or *because of your own illness.* Many people who have heard of this provision still believe, perhaps because of the word "family" in the title, that it applies only to those caring for a sick relative. As we have stressed previously, this is not the case. It can be used to care for yourself, as well as to care for others, and therefore is an important resource for cancer patients and survivors to be aware of. It should be noted that this form of leave only applies if your employer has 50 or more employees, and is in general *unpaid.* You may, however, be able to use paid sick or vacation days that you have accrued. In most cases this provision assures you 12 weeks of leave, which may be used at one time, or broken up into different periods. While you are on FMLA, your employer is obligated to continue your health coverage.

FMLA (Family and Medical Leave Act)

Law passed by congress in 1993 stating that in most cases employers must grant an employee up to 12 work weeks of unpaid leave during any 12-month period, in order to care for an immediate family member, or because of their own serious health condition.

PART FIVE

Too Young for Cancer

I had cancer when I was 8 years old. Now when I see a doctor I sometimes leave that out, because it was so long ago. That's okay, right?

When I got my diagnosis, I had to leave college and move back in with my parents. Can I ever really get back on track?

I'm 25 years old and finished treatment for testicular cancer last year. Now I feel out of sync with other people my own age. How do I handle this "generation gap?"

More . . .

Always tell a new doctor that you had cancer, even if it was long ago.

65. I am 28 years old. I had cancer when I was 8 years old. Now when I see a doctor I sometimes leave that out, because it was so long ago. That's okay, right?

Wrong! It's great that your illness is in the past and that you feel that you've moved on. But your doctors do need to know about your cancer history. Although it sounds like your treatment was curative and that you are now disease-free, that same treatment may have implications for your health in the future. Certain types of chemotherapy, radiation, and surgery can put you at risk for problems—some very minor, and some more serious. The more your doctor knows about your treatment, the more help she can be in helping you to stay healthy. Beth Whittam, Nurse Practioner in the Program for Adult Survivors of Pediatric Cancers at Memorial Sloan-Kettering Cancer Center reminds us that the optimum circumstance is for you to find out *exactly* what kind(s) of treatment you received—including doses of chemotherapy and number of rads of radiation. This way your doctor can home in on what you both want to look out for as time goes by, and what kind of tests and scans may be needed to follow you. Though it may be hard to hear, the fact is that some secondary effects of treatment often don't show up until 20 or 30 years later. Your history of cancer and its treatment remain an important factor in your care throughout your lifetime.

So, even if you are feeling well and not experiencing any symptoms at all, it is still vital that you tell your health care provider about your childhood cancer. As Whittam again reminds us, "Many secondary problems can be treated, or even prevented, if they are discovered early."

66. When I got my diagnosis, I had to leave college and move back in with my parents. I missed a year of school, can't graduate with my class, and frankly feel like a huge baby for living at home. Can I ever really get back on track?

Cancer is a disruptive illness whenever it occurs. But perhaps the most disruptive time to receive a diagnosis is during young adulthood. Just as you're in the process of moving out and making a life of your own, pursuing advanced education or building a career, you are derailed by illness. Many young survivors describe this need to leave their peer group and return to their childhood home as an especially frustrating injury, added to the insult of cancer. Being at home can be tough in many ways. Although we all need our families when we hit tough times, for young adults being at home can feel like the proverbial two steps back. Not only are they less independent, but some find that parents and other family members behave in a way that feels overprotective, even smothering. "I know my mom is only worried, because she loves me. But does she actually think that I need someone to tell me to put on a sweater when it's cold?" asks Tim. This kind of close scrutiny can be frustrating at a time when you have been on your own for a while.

As we have mentioned earlier, another factor that makes young patients feel confused and isolated is being treated in areas of the hospital where they are the only ones their age. Some Hodgkin's patients may be hospitalized on a pediatric floor, intensifying the feeling of being a "huge baby." Others may have a roommate in his seventies, causing the young adult patient to wonder if having cancer means that he is now elderly himself. These struggles only serve as a concrete reminder of how hard it is to find your place as a young adult with cancer.

It is not only challenging to be part of the medical world as a young patient. Other parts of the picture are also tough to deal with, as we've noted previously. At times you may feel that you are literally living in a different world from that of the friends you left behind at school. It is also deeply frustrating to step off a well-planned educational path into what can seem like the limbo of treatment and recovery.

There is no easy answer to reclaiming your place in a world you've lost touch with. It will take time and effort, and will involve painful moments, like watching friends graduate and knowing that you might have done so with them, if it hadn't been for your illness. But, as hard as it may be to believe, the cancer experience doesn't have to be only about friends lost and journeys interrupted. It can also be about new friends found, and new journeys begun. Time and again we have seen this happen, whether in camping programs or in other activities that enable you to meet other young adults with cancer.

Throughout this book, we stress the importance of such support organizations in helping cancer patients to feel less isolated and better understood. Such resources are perhaps most important for people like you. When you leave your school friends, and spend most of your time in the medical world, it's easy to feel alone. We can't stress enough that this is not the case. More and more, young adult cancer patients have their own programs and networks. They no longer need to use a "one size fits all" system of support, where they may be thrown into groups with those much older or much younger than they are. Because young adults are more familiar with technology than any other age group, many of these programs are online. We hope that you'll take a look at our list of resources in the back of the book and choose those that seem right for you.

67. I'm 25 years old and finished treatment for testicular cancer last year. Now I feel out of sync with other people my own age—almost like I'm much older than they are. Some of the stuff they do frankly seems kind of dumb to me, like staying out all night, smoking, or getting drunk. How do I handle this "generation gap?"

Over time, the "generation gap" between you and your peers will begin to close.

You are raising an issue that we hear about in every young adult meeting we have.

The out-of-sync feeling certainly begins the minute a young person receives their diagnosis; after all, most people don't get life-threatening illness until they are much older. The feeling may only intensify when the person is in the hospital. As we've noted, sometimes they may find themselves the oldest one on a pediatric ward, surrounded by toys, teddy bears, and brightly colored clowns on the walls. Others may attend a local support group, only to find that the other participants are all their grandparents' age. In both these cases, the young adult patient might well ask, "What am I doing here?"

Once they move into survivorship, they encounter the kind of situation you describe. After going through such a deeply challenging and life-altering experience, it may be hard to take up the identity of a carefree college student or young professional. For these groups, life is still very much about having fun, and celebrating youth, energy and good health. Young adults also tend to have a feeling of invulnerability— believing that they never will, or could be, ill. This is part of what smoking and drinking is about, after all. Clearly, those who have had a life-threatening illness will not share that feeling of being invulnerable. Understandably, you will not want to take risks with your health. And, yes, that is a big

Too Young for Cancer

difference between you and your peers, and one that can't be ignored.

It would be wrong to tell you that your changed feelings won't get in the way of socializing with people your age at times. It is simply a fact of life that your cancer experience has changed the way you feel about things. But what we also hear is that young people who've had cancer often win the admiration of their peers. In some ways they *are* seen as older, and so are valued for their perceived wisdom and maturity.

We can almost hear you saying that you don't just want to be wise—you want to have fun! But of course, there are still many activities that you can participate in—movies, dinners out (with or without a cocktail or glass of wine), or going to a ball game. And, believe it or not, eventually some of your peers will catch up with you in maturity and a more philosophical view of life.

68. I lost my fertility as a result of my cancer treatment. Now a lot of my friends are having babies. It's really painful for me to be at all those showers. But isn't it rude not to go?

It sounds like you want very much to be a good friend, and celebrate the joy of those around you. But most survivors who attend our discussion groups agree that the usual rules of etiquette must be modified after cancer. There are many things that may prevent survivors from wanting to participate in a given event—fatigue, difficulty traveling, problems with eating, or emotional issues. For you, attendance at a baby shower isn't a simple social event. It is a painful reminder of a deep loss. You—and your friends—should take that into account, and cut you a little slack. Those who truly care for you are likely to understand.

You don't need to actually be present at a shower, however, to show that you care. You can send a gift, or, if shopping for a gift is also too painful, order a bouquet of flowers to be delivered on the day of the shower for everyone to enjoy.

Is there one close and trusted person that you could talk openly with about your feelings here? Then you can decide how much you want to share with others. It is all right to say, "I am so happy for you, but a baby-centered event would be hard for me right now." Or, you could keep your reasons private, and simply say that you're sorry you can't make it that day, but send your very best wishes.

PART SIX

Maintaining Your Health

I've heard that it's important to have a "positive attitude" in order to stay well. But sometimes when life is challenging it's hard to feel positive. Does this mean I'll be more likely to get cancer again?

Everything I read about cancer stresses the importance of diet, so I made a lot of changes in the way I eat. Am I going to be sick again if I don't stick to the right diet?

So what *can* I do to remain free of cancer?

More . . .

Don't pressure yourself to think positively all the time; it just isn't realistic.

69. I've heard that it's important to have a "positive attitude" in order to stay well. But sometimes when life is challenging it's hard to feel positive. Does this mean I'll be more likely to get cancer again?

Many survivors raise this question. Anyone who has had cancer wants to do whatever they can to stay healthy, and if they hear that a positive attitude will do this, they naturally try to adopt one. But this can be challenging, especially when one is coping with the multiple life changes that may accompany cancer, dealing with after-effects of treatment, and worrying about the future. We often hear that the pressure to stay positive merely *adds* stress to the life of a survivor—which is the last thing you want!

Jimmie Holland, MD, who holds the Wayne E. Chapman Chair in Psychiatric Oncology at Memorial Sloan-Kettering Cancer Center, often speaks of what she calls "the tyranny of positive thinking." She has seen all too often how survivors berate and frighten themselves during those times that they struggle to feel "up."

After a powerful and life-changing experience, it is simply not possible to be on an even keel all the time. While no one would make the claim that a hopeless or despairing attitude is the key to a happy life (with or without cancer), it isn't realistic to expect yourself to look on the sunny side every minute of every day, no matter what. The best way to be positive, without being "tyrannized," is to remain open to joyful moments as they come.

70. I am cancer free and want to stay that way. Everything I read about cancer stresses the importance of diet, so I made a lot of changes in the way I eat. I started to buy only organic food, to make fresh juices each day, and to eat lots fruit and vegetables. But I can't always get organic products—and when I do, they're expensive. And some days I don't have time to juice. Am I going to be sick again if I don't stick to the right diet?

The experience of illness can make us feel helpless and out of control. This can be particularly pronounced in cancer, not only because it is life-threatening, but because it often appears with few or no symptoms; this gives it a sneaky quality that other diseases may not have. After an out-of-control experience, it's natural to want to get that control back in any way we can. Some people find themselves doing this in ways that have a superstitious quality ("If I'm more patient with my elderly mother, then I won't get sick again.") Others seek information, as you have done, about factors that contribute to illness and to wellness. Much of what you've learned is based on real scientific data, and it obviously doesn't constitute superstitious thinking. But as real as this information may be, it sounds like you may be using it to set impossible goals—and then feeling anxious when you cannot meet them. As Donald Garrity, RD, CDN, nutrition counselor at the Integrative Medicine Service of Memorial Sloan-Kettering Cancer reminds us, "It's fairly well accepted that a diet that emphasizes fruits, vegetables, whole grains, and lean meats contributes to better overall health. But it can be hard to make a series of major dietary changes all at once. Why don't you start with small steps that take you towards your goal of healthy eating? Each person has to decide for himself how much he or she wants to alter his diet, and then work up to that point gradually. This is the best way to stay on course, without getting overly stressed out about what you eat."

71. So *what* can *I do to remain free of cancer?*

Wouldn't it be great if there were a "magic bullet," that would assure that you wouldn't get cancer again. This kind of guarantee is something that everyone wishes for, whether they have been sick or not. Because so many people fear cancer—and this fear may be heightened for those who have already been sick—it can be frustrating that the question of cause and cure is so often unanswerable. But living with this type of uncertainty does become easier over time.

Still, there are some basic guidelines that may assist the cancer survivor in remaining healthy. Nancy Houlihan, clinical nurse specialist at the Cancer Survivorship Program of Memorial Sloan-Kettering Cancer Center reminds us that one important step is to get screened for types of cancer other than the one for which you're being followed. You should be sure to have a colonoscopy, as well as a mammogram if you're a woman, and a **PSA blood test** (to detect prostate cancer), if you're male. Naturally, it is wise to stop smoking or not to start, to limit alcohol intake, keep your weight down, and exercise as often as possible, preferably engaging in weight-bearing activity.

PSA blood test

Prostate-Specific Antigen test, administered to men to measure the level of a tumor marker for prostate cancer in the blood.

Again, since cancer is something everyone worries about, we all hear a lot on the news about what contributes to it and how it can be prevented. During the many years we've worked in this field, we have seen recommendations come and go, whether they involved coffee, soy products, or vitamins. The hype surrounding these substances is something we have learned over time to tune out, realizing that in many cases the jury will be out on the issue for many years to come.

But even as you pursue the sensible goals recommended above, it is important to remember that being preoccupied with your health is not a way of achieving a sense of well-being. Follow the guidelines suggested by your medical team, and then . . . breathe.

72. I want to return to work, volunteering, and the PTA. But I've heard that stress can cause cancer. If I do too much, will it make me sick?

While working with cancer survivors to achieve the best possible quality of life, we often wonder if the worst stressor that they face is worrying about stress!

No one can say for sure whether stress plays a role in developing cancer.

Although this sounds like a joke, there is a great deal of truth to it. It's understandable for survivors to want to remain well, and to be willing to do whatever is required to maintain their health. Many hear, as you do, that stress plays a role in the development or recurrence of cancer. The truth is that the medical jury is out on this issue, but we certainly agree that minimizing stress is a good idea for anyone. If you've been through the rigors of cancer treatment, you are especially deserving of a life that is free of excessive demands. And staying as free of negative stress is important in order to function at your best—including keeping up with medical tests and appointments. But be aware that the jury is still out on how much stress contributes to the development of cancer, with early science indicating little or no connection.

So the answer here is really up to you. It is not a question of excessive activity making you sick again. It's a question of how much you *want* to do. If keeping busy and contributing your time to activities you care about is meaningful to you, there isn't a reason in the world you shouldn't continue to do so. There is even such a thing as "good" stress—a level of excitement and involvement that contributes to our well being. But if fatigue is an issue, or if, like many survivors, you find that your priorities have changed, you may want to limit the number of things you agree to do. The important thing is that you are in charge here.

Post-treatment fatigue is normal, but if you're worried, then check with your doctor.

73. My treatment ended over a year ago. But I still feel really, really tired. Sometimes doing the simplest thing wipes me out. I am taking a nap nearly every day. Is there something wrong with me?

Naturally, when you have any troubling symptom, the first thing to do is check in with your health care team. It is important to rule out any underlying symptom, such as anemia, which could be causing your fatigue. And of course, finding a clear contributing factor means that treatment (and relief) can be offered.

But once your physician or nurse has ruled out any clear health issue, you may want to know that one of the most common complaints we hear from new survivors is ongoing fatigue. It is hard to say how long this may last, because it differs from person to person, but know that you are not alone with this troubling symptom.

Let's let some survivors comment:

Eliza: *It's so frustrating! If I do something during the day, I have to stay in and rest in the evening. If I have evening plans, I have to rest all day!*

Luis: *The only way to describe this feeling is to tell you that the other day I was crossing the street. Right in the middle I felt so tired, I didn't think I would make it to the other side, I couldn't believe it when I actually stepped onto the curb.*

In addition to being disappointing and disabling, this pervasive post-treatment fatigue can also be frightening. Many survivors become understandably concerned that their cancer has returned—or was never successfully treated. In the vast majority of cases, this is not what is going on.

Most health practitioners suggest that you cope with fatigue in the following ways: First, take note of which times of the day you seem to have the most energy, and try to plan any around that "peak time." Secondly, learn to prioritize, deciding which activities are most meaningful to you, and skipping those which don't matter as much. As we discuss throughout the book, this is something that many survivors find themselves doing in any case.

Many health food and other stores offer products and substances which claim to "increase energy." Be cautious in using such things, and be sure to check with your doctor before doing so. If you want to check on the usefulness or safety of herbs and botanicals you can log onto the website *About Herbs, Botanicals & Other Products* available at: http://www.mskcc.org/mskcc/html/11570.cfm.

Dave comments:

I think the lesson I learned is that cancer can have a debilitating effect on one's life, degrading both physical and mental well being. However, the human body is a powerful mechanism that can rise to and overcome many challenges. I have always been physically active and have played competitive racquetball most of my life. I was relieved when my treatment was completed, but I did feel that I was weaker, older, and slower. I continued to workout and play competitively, but my performance was still less than par and I resigned myself to having to live with a lower level of performance. About ten months after my last procedure I began to see some improvement, and now, after fourteen months have passed, I feel that I am stronger than before I was diagnosed.

74. About halfway through my chemotherapy, I began to have a funny feeling in my hands and feet—a tingling, numb sensation. I finished up two months ago, but still feel it. Could it be connected with my treatment?

Peripheral neuropathy

Nerve damage in the extremities that may cause numbness, tingling, or weakness.

It sounds like you're describing something called **peripheral neuropathy.** This is a condition that comes about when certain nerves (those controlling touch and temperature, as well as those that control movement), have been damaged. There are a number of things that can cause this damage, including some illnesses, alcohol abuse, or vitamin deficiencies. But it is not uncommon for people who have been treated for cancer to develop this condition as a result of their treatment. Both surgery and radiation can damage nerves, but most often the problem is caused by chemotherapy. The list of agents that may cause this troubling side effect is a long one; check with your doctor to learn whether the type of chemotherapy that you were on is among them. And of course, discuss your overall condition with your doctor in order to determine whether another factor may be involved.

In some cases, people have nerve pain, as well as the numbness and tingling you describe. This pain can usually be treated. Sometimes the treatment may include drugs usually used to combat depression. If your medical team suggests them, this does *not* mean they think you are imagining your distress! Such medications are useful because they affect the membrane around the nerves. But in most cases, when pain is not the primary issue, there is no really effective treatment for neuropathy.

It is important to be aware of any long-term effects that your treatment might cause.

Sometimes doctors neglect to mention peripheral neuropathy, leaving patients and survivors very anxious when they note new and uncomfortable sensations. And, unfortunately, when people *do* bring it up to their health care team, they may find that it is dismissed as simply the unpleasant price of treatment. But we hope that your doctor can reassure you that this symptom does not mean your disease has spread or recurred; it is a common side effect, and not a new illness.

Although some people find that their neuropathy is lasting, for most people, it will diminish over time.

75. Ever since my chemo finished, I've noticed that I'm very forgetful and "spacey." I lose my keys, leave things burning on the stove, and once even forgot to pick up my son at school! Am I losing my mind?

Absolutely not. What you are experiencing is something that many survivors have been describing for years. In fact, this phenomenon is so common that survivors have coined a term for it—**chemo brain.** And it is now getting serious attention from physicians and researchers.

Ever since we began offering support services to cancer patients, starting 20 years ago, we have heard survivors mention distressing symptoms, such as those you describe. As one woman put it "I feel like I've lost my mind, or at least misplaced it, along with my car keys." No one can say who first coined the term "chemo brain," but it soon caught on like wildfire because it described something shared by so many. Many patients and survivors expressed frustration at being told by their doctors that there was no such thing. (This was, incidentally, an example of how valuable support groups can be; it meant a great deal to survivors to find their feelings and perceptions validated by others.) The doctors themselves are not to blame for this stance, since there was little or no research on the phenomenon their patients were describing. But as patients become more vocal, assertive, and proactive over the years, the scientific world began to take notice. Studies have shown that nearly all people treated with chemotherapy suffer some form of short-term memory loss. In other words, chemo brain is real.

Chemo brain

A term coined by cancer survivors to describe problems with memory loss and concentration following chemotherapy treatment.

But it is still hard for researchers to know just what causes it because there are so many complicating factors. We know that treatment often causes fatigue, which can itself impair one's thinking. So can treatment-related anemia. For women, chemotherapy often leads to an abrupt entry into menopause, leading doctors to wonder if cognitive problems may really be a series of "senior moments" for these patients. Depression, too, can cause mental confusion. Finally, it is difficult to measure thinking problems in a person if you don't know what his thinking was like before.

Still, even as the scientific world continues to grapple with questions about chemo brain, so do patients. Doctors are beginning to respond by prescribing medications that offer some relief, such as those given for attention-deficit disorder, or to help people with a sleeping disorder called narcolepsy stay awake. Sometimes antidepressant medication offers a little help. And, of course, it can be a relief just to have your difficulties acknowledged, which most health care professionals do at this point.

Finally, take hope in the fact that, for most people, this condition clears up to a great degree over time; only a small minority of survivors report an ongoing problem with focus and memory. Until then, try not to panic, or worse, to be angry with yourself when you have trouble—and know that you are not alone.

76. I've been cancer-free for many years. Recently, I moved, and don't see my surgeon or oncologist any more. Who do I see now for my follow up care?

There are many ways that you can handle this common dilemma. First you can call the doctors who treated you in the first place and ask them for a referral to a doctor near you. This is a good first step because they know your medical history and would be able to make the most appropriate referral to an oncologist or cancer specialist that best suits your current needs. If that first step doesn't work, the second way to handle this would be to contact the National Cancer Institute's (NCI) Cancer Information Service (800-4-CANCER) and ask them who they recommend for your follow up care. They should have a listing of all the NCI-designated cancer centers in the country and again from there you could get a referral in your area.

The other possibility is to discuss this with your internist and see if she has any recommendations for oncologists or surgeons. Another thing you can do is contact your nearest **teaching hospital,** where you can locate doctors who have a faculty practice (private office). Such physicians have the advantage of being part of the hospital setting with all the resources that accompany it, such as current research and developments in many aspects of care as well as clinical trials.

The main thing to remember it is important to maintain follow up to your care no matter how many years you have been away from treatment.

Teaching hospital

Medical facility that not only provides primary medical care, but also offers experimental or unique treatments and conducts research.

77. I am so freaked out! On my most recent medical visit, the nurse mentioned there could be "late effects" of my treatment. I thought all this was behind me. What did she mean?

It would be great if cancer was an experience with a clear beginning, middle, and end. But unfortunately, treatment does have implications for your health in the future. The most important thing to remember is that any doctor who sees you during your lifetime should be aware of your cancer history, so that he or she can be on the alert for any problem you may have, and intervene as early as possible.

For a better understanding of what late effects of treatment may be, let's turn again to survivorship nurse Nancy Houlihan who explains:

Late effects are conditions that may occur years after treatment is complete. Most oncologists will inform you about late effects to be aware of, though some will not want to burden you with this information early on in your survivorship. This may be especially true if you were treated as a child, because we didn't know as much about the long-term effects of treatment years ago.

One possible late effect is damage to the heart caused by some chemotherapy drugs. Again, this may not turn up until long after your treatment is over, so it is helpful for both you and any doctor you see to be aware of the kind of chemotherapy you have had. Radiation too, may cause heart problems, or damage to the lungs.

Finally, it is also the case that some types of chemotherapy and radiation can cause second cancers. Being watched carefully in an ongoing way will make sure that any problem you may have is caught early.

Although it's important to be aware of the possibility of late effects of treatment, it should not dominate your life. Remember, there wouldn't *be* any late effects, if your cancer hadn't been successfully treated. Bear this in mind, and keep your worries about long-term problems in balance with the good news of your current state of wellness.

PART SEVEN

Sex, Intimacy, and Fertility

My partner was great during the treatment for endometrial cancer. Now that it's been a few months, it seems like she's avoiding sex. Does she find me less attractive now?

When should I tell someone I'm dating that I've had cancer?

But if I wait too long to tell someone about my history, aren't I being dishonest?

More . . .

78. My partner was great during the treatment for endometrial cancer. Now that it's been a few months, it seems like she's working later than usual, doesn't want to talk when she gets home, and just seems kind of disconnected. We have zero intimate contact, and frankly I feel that she's avoiding sex. Does she find me less attractive now?

So—just when you need to be reassured of your worth and attractiveness, your partner seems more far away than ever. This is definitely a hard place for you to be. But it would be premature to make any assumptions about what's going on between you, without considering a few things.

Many partners tell us that they are deeply confused about how to behave once their loved one has gone through cancer treatment. They talk primarily about two issues. One worry they express is their feeling that their own wishes and desires should be put on the back burner, and the focus placed only on the comfort of the person who has been ill. "I feel like it would be wrong to let her know I want sex," says Ed, who had been married to Liz for 25 years when her breast cancer was diagnosed. "She has so many other things to worry about. Wouldn't it be selfish of me to ask for what I want?"

Another major worry among partners, especially when the cancer affected a part of the body directly involved in sexual activity, is that they will hurt the person who has been ill. We have often been asked whether it's all right to touch a breast that has been radiated or reconstructed. Can the skin be damaged by too much friction? Could the implant burst?

Don't assume that your partner is less interested in you just because she isn't showing an interest in sexual activity now. Just like you, she may be making a great number of assumptions about your wishes or concerns. While it's hard to risk an open conversation when you're feeling fearful and insecure, that is the only thing that can clear up any misconceptions you or your partner may have. It may also turn out that she has some questions that your nurse or doctor could address, helping her to feel more comfortable about getting close. Just as you are learning about your own feelings, and your own body, so is your partner. It can be very helpful to talk about them together.

79. When should I tell someone I'm dating that I've had cancer? If I tell them before they get to know me, I'm afraid they'll be scared and run away. But if I wait longer, I'll feel dishonest. What should I do?

We often say that there is no right time to tell someone of your cancer history; most people sense when the time is right. But—there are two wrong times. One is obviously when you first meet someone, and they haven't had a chance to learn anything about you. This is what one young survivor called the "Hello, I had cancer" introduction. Why should the only thing they know be that you are a cancer survivor? In fact, a person might wonder why you raised such an intimate issue so early in the game.

The other time that we don't advise sharing your cancer story is when you are about to become intimate sexually. This is a "set up" that isn't fair to you *or* your partner. How would you feel if someone you were dating shared something very important, something you wanted to reflect on and digest, just as you were about to go to bed? Unfortunately, survivors sometimes choose this time, in order to explain scars, discoloration, or other body changes. But again, not giving the other person time to absorb this information sets you both up for awkwardness or hurt. It could be that you mistake someone's surprise for distaste or rejection; we have seen this happen more than once. And if the other person *does* have second thoughts about being involved with you after learning about your cancer, you have put yourself in a needlessly vulnerable position.

You will note that we refer to your cancer experience as an intimate issue—rather than a secret, or worse, a crime to be confessed. We think it makes a real difference if you can view it this way, too. Many people tell us that cancer makes them feel like "damaged goods." Naturally this feeling leads them to believe they have something to apologize for. But remember—your cancer also makes you the person you are now. Perhaps you have grown or become more understanding of others through having cancer. Maybe you are stronger, wiser, and less superficial than people who have never been challenged in this way. The way that you think about yourself and your cancer will come across to others. If you are ashamed or apologetic, others will sense that.

We suggest that you wait as long to discuss your cancer history as you would to share any other personal and intimate information—family problems, money issues, sexual habits, the contents of your journal, and many others.

When dating someone new, don't feel pressure to "confess" that you had cancer.

80. But if I wait too long to tell someone about my history, aren't I being dishonest?

Again, your question suggests that you feel you have something to "confess," and that not doing so is immoral or unfair. There is, of course, some truth in this. If you and your partner are planning a life together, and you have left out an important part of who you are, that is indeed dishonest.

But most people who ask these questions are nowhere near that place. They are simply so anxious about the other person's reaction that they want to hasten the process. This is understandable. But the reason to talk sooner rather than later is not to avoid cheating another person—it's to avoid cheating *yourself*. It is easy to focus so much on the other guy that you leave yourself out of the equation. We find it is most helpful not to think of being fair to the other person, but of being fair to *you*. You don't deserve to become invested in someone who may not be understanding or accepting of your health history. You *do* deserve to have the information about what this person can handle—after all, won't that be important to you, in planning a life together? Would you want to be with someone who judged you for having cancer, or who was so afraid of it they couldn't discuss it with you?

Finally, people who've had cancer often focus so much on their own discomfort about this, that they assume that no one else has any worries or "flaws." Remember, everyone has a history of some kind. They may have health or family issues that they are concerned about sharing. It can be helpful if you don't idealize the other person, and remember that he or she isn't perfect either.

81. If I tell a prospective partner about my cancer history, will the person still want to go out with me?

The only fair answer to this is: maybe yes, and maybe no. It would be wrong to tell you that you will never meet someone who is scared or put off by the fact that you had cancer. As we all know, this is a frightening illness, and there are people who are so anxious that they can't face it at all. This may be because of superstition or misinformation, or because they may have had a painful experience with cancer that hit close to home. (Especially if this happened before there were as many treatment options as there are now.) You are not responsible for other people's feelings. When someone is fearful or anxious about your cancer history, try to remember that this has nothing to do with you as a person; it is about their limitation, not yours. (This is a shame, because, not only will they miss out on meeting some great people—but what will they do if someone already close should become ill? Or if they must face cancer themselves?) We know that it may seem easy for us to tell you not to be bothered by what is, after all, a type of rejection. But it can help to know at the outset that this may happen. But it won't happen with everyone, and you do have some influence on the reactions of others. Much depends upon how and when you share your history. We'll discuss that as we respond to the following questions.

82. I am a single man and I have survived cancer a couple of years. I used to meet prospective partners through my gym, but everyone there is in such great shape, and looks so healthy. I'm afraid that if I meet a new guy, and he sees my scars—not to mention how quickly I tire out—he won't be interested. How do I deal with people's reactions to my "imperfect" body?

It is always difficult to deal with physical changes, even if they're not in a form that's visible to others. When changes are apparent to others, the challenge can be even greater.

You describe your gym as a place that's not just about fitness, but is also a social venue. In a gym, that social component may indeed have a lot to do with how people look, or with how strong or capable they are—and we know that both these things can change after a cancer experience.

As we reiterate throughout this book, much of your interaction with others depends on your own attitude. If you are ashamed of your body or of having gone through cancer, then you may behave in a withdrawn or unavailable way. This will certainly influence how others respond to you. We've seen many survivors who are open and comfortable about bodily changes—which may be scars, radiation tattoos, or even missing limbs—connect with others in a positive way. Their own comfort level helps others to be comfortable too.

In fact, for many of these people, the changes, along with an "open door" attitude, actually help them to connect, as others ask about them, or say "Hey, we've missed you around here? What's been going on?" One young woman, Tara, who walked with a cane, invented something she called "the dance of the seven veils." Let's let her describe it:

When I meet a new person, and they ask about my cane, I respond that I'm having a problem with my hip, but I'm fine and dealing with it. If I see that person again, I may say 'I had some surgery last year.' Finally, if we're getting close, I tell the whole story. I feel like this keeps me in control. And adds a layer of mystery!

But there is something else to add here: Many people who have been through cancer describe changes that go far deeper than altered appearance. Some say that their priorities are different, and that this alters their choice of friends and partners. Although it may have been important at one time to find someone with movie-star looks (and to be very good-looking oneself) it may now seem more meaningful to find someone who is trustworthy, kind, loyal, a good conversationalist—even if he or she wouldn't make the cover of a magazine.

Finally, everyone is imperfect in some way. Don't assume that you are the only person at the gym who is struggling—even if your struggle is more visible.

83. The treatment for my prostate cancer left me unable to have an erection, despite the medication my doctor gave me for erectile dysfunction. I'm a divorced guy who would really like to remarry. I guess this puts the lid on my chances, right?

The short answer is: no. But let's discuss your situation in more depth.

Sex, Intimacy, and Fertility

As we know, cancer patients are increasingly asking not only to survive their disease, but also to have a satisfying quality of life when treatment ends. This is certainly at the heart of your question. Not only do you want to gain pleasure from sex, but also you want to find a partner with whom you can be intimate—and who will experience pleasure as well. There is no reason that this should not happen, whether you become able to maintain an erection or not. But first, let's discuss your options.

First of all, we hope you've consulted a urologist who specializes in erectile dysfunction. There are more and more doctors who do so, and you should certainly see one. If you've already tried oral medication, he or she may want to discuss other treatments. The most likely medication he would suggest next is alprostadil, given either by injection into the penis, or by suppository. Like oral medication, the way that alprostadil works is by increasing blood flow, throughout the body. Naturally, this affects the penis. The injection provides an erection sufficient for intercourse in about 80% of cases, a higher success rate than suppositories, which work in 30 to 40% of cases, when placed into the opening at the tip of the penis. The medication will begin to work within five to twenty minutes; the erection will last about an hour. There are certain precautions with alprostadil, which you should discuss with your doctor.

If injections or suppositories don't work for you, another option is a penile prosthesis. This may take the form of pliable rods surgically implanted in the penis. In this case, the penis is always partially rigid; the position must just be adjusted in order to have intercourse. A more popular choice now is an inflatable device, which operates on a hydraulic principle. This allows a man to have an erection when he chooses, and is more natural. Most men who use this option rate it highly, and say they still have sensation, as well as orgasms.

But your question also brings to mind an episode that occurred in one of our group meetings on dating after cancer. Although men were in the minority in the group, there was one who spoke frequently, offering advice and encouragement to other members. He assured the women in the meeting that they remained attractive and that they appeared to have a great deal to offer. He passed his handkerchief to one woman who shed some tears after talking about her own fears about dating again. Shortly before the end of the group, this man said that he knew no woman could be interested in him. Although he and his doctor had tried many remedies, he was unable to maintain an erection. For this reason, he said, it was unlikely that anyone would want more than a couple of dates with him. "After all," he said, "if a woman has a choice between good sex and a nice sensitive guy, she's going to go for the sex, right?" With no prompting, a chorus of female voices shouted "Wrong!" in unison. As the group dissolved in laughter, one woman said "Hey—I practically fell in love with you already! Kindness and consideration are my number one requirements in a man." The other women all nodded.

Although we understand that you want the fullest sex life possible, bear in mind that many other qualities are valuable to the opposite sex. Perhaps more than you think.

84. My partner is as loving as ever since I finished treatment. But I have no interest in sexual activity now. What's wrong with me?

It is rare for the partner of a cancer survivor to cease valuing that person, or to stop wanting to remain connected sexually. But for the survivor, the wish to connect through sexual activity may change. There are many reasons for this. Let's look at some of them.

Sometimes cancer treatment brings about functional changes. For men who have been treated for prostate cancer, it is

Cancer may change your interest in sex, or your response to it, for a wide variety of reasons.

sometimes difficult to have or maintain an erection. While such problems can often be addressed with medication, this can still cause the survivor to feel anxious about performance. Many men say they don't initiate intimate contact because they don't want to start something they can't finish. This may in turn lead their partner to feel unwanted or rejected. This sequence can lead to a cycle of misunderstanding and distance. It's true that a part of the relationship has been profoundly changed, and this loss must be acknowledged, but it is also possible to find many ways to remain close and connected. It's even possible to learn to be sexual in new and different ways; it is not always important for intercourse to occur. In a meeting of survivors that included both men and women, a survivor of prostate cancer said that he had "nothing to offer a woman" besides kissing, holding hands, and caressing. There was a lot of laughter when a chorus of women answered in unison, "Sounds great to me!"

Women, too, may find their sexual functioning has been affected by treatment. Surgery and chemotherapy both can plunge a woman into menopause suddenly, instead of permitting the natural process that might take place over a number of years. Vaginal dryness and discomfort can make sexual activity unpleasant, even painful. Getting used to these changes and learning the best way to address them will take time. Your doctor or nurse should be able to recommend a number of commercial products that can be helpful (including some you may already have around the house, like olive oil). Being in menopause may also mean a lowered libido for many—but not all—women. Many women say that it simply takes longer for them to "warm up" than it did before. Touching, stroking, and massaging can make a difference here. Some people find that erotic books or movies can be helpful.

But even if functional changes have not occurred, many cancer survivors say that sex is not the first—or second, or third—thing on their minds.

Laura, a 34-year-old cancer survivor of thyroid cancer says:

When your life is threatened, it's like the house is on fire. All you want to do is put out the fire—nothing else matters. During my treatment, and for a long time afterward, all I could focus on was my health.

Danny, a 38-year-old brain tumor survivor adds:

I know this sounds crazy, but I'm still working out a lot of the 'leftovers' of treatment. After I've been on the phone with my insurance company for three hours, trying to get them to pay for my prescription meds, I'm not exactly in a romantic mood.

For these reasons and many others, it may take time for a survivor's sex life to get back on track. And that track may not look or feel just as it did before. Talking openly about all this with a partner can help them to see that they are not being rejected, just that you need some time and understanding.

85. When I had cancer, my wife had to do everything for me. She drove me to and from treatments, made me special foods, and took care of all the bills and banking. Now that treatment is over, I feel that the balance in our marriage is off. How do I get back to being the strong guy she can lean on?

It's not surprising that you feel that something in your marriage has shifted. In most partnerships, tasks are divided, with each partner taking care of what he or she does best. When one person becomes too sick to do his half, the other usually picks up the slack. It sounds like this is what has happened with you and your wife, leaving you feeling like you're not holding up your end of the bargain. In some ways, that may be true. But there are other aspects of a partnership, too—subtler agreements that may be unspoken. One of those is that, if one partner needs help for a time, the other will be there to pitch in. Have you asked yourself if you would have done the same if your wife had been the one who was sick? You almost certainly would have. Another thing to consider is what really constitutes a partnership. After all, it's not just about shared tasks. It is also about caring for and about the other person, understanding them, and being in their corner. This is something you have probably continued to do, even when sick. It is an important way of being someone that your wife can lean on.

Another way of looking at the crisis of cancer is that it allows the well partner to discover strengths and abilities they may not have been aware of. One woman spoke with pride of all that she learned by taking over some of the roles that had formerly been filled by her husband. She said shyly, "Do you know that I had never really read a map before? That was always Harvey's job. It sounds silly, but I feel so good about it!" This doesn't mean that your importance to your wife is diminished, only that she may feel better about herself, which is good for both of you.

Be patient. It may take time for you to resume roles that had to be set aside when you were on treatment. And it may also be that those roles look somewhat different now. As we said earlier, your wife may want to hold on to some of the tasks she took on, finding that they are satisfying to her. You may find that you have a wish to do things differently yourself. It will take some time for this to shake out and become clearer.

Finally, if your wife is feeling depleted or wrung out by all that she has taken on, and needs a break, you can tell her that you're now able to do much more than before, and suggest that she visit a friend in another city, or go to a spa for a break. Doing so will let you both know that you are on the road to recovery.

86. I don't see how anyone could want to see my scarred body. Isn't it best just to accept that the sexual part of my life is over, and move on?

It sounds like you're making up others' minds for them. This is understandable, because people who have had cancer (or other illnesses or body changes) are often afraid that they are no longer desirable. Your question makes it sound like you don't have a partner at the moment, so naturally this is of concern to you. (This concern obviously takes a different form for those with partners, and we address that issue elsewhere.) But let's talk about you. There are a few things to remember here.

First, we can all be sexual beings, no matter what we look like, assuming that this is important to you. If you were interested in sexual feelings and activity before having cancer, there is no reason you shouldn't continue to find this part of life meaningful. Many survivors feel that the best way to get back into sexual activity is on their own, through masturbation. Sometimes the effects of treatment require that you get to know your body and its responses in a new way. A lot of people feel that doing this exploration on their own prepares them to communicate their needs to others. If you choose not to go beyond finding pleasure on your own, that is certainly your decision, and up to no one but you.

Secondly, you are assuming that everyone who is seeking a partner requires that that person be perfect. It's certainly true that some people judge others primarily by their appearance—but just as many do not. We can't help wondering whether your cancer experience may have added a deeper dimension to the person you are. Maybe you want to look for someone else who shares that kind of depth and complexity.

Finally, even if your body bears some "battle scars," there are no doubt parts of you that remain very attractive—such as

It takes time for partners to return to the sexual closeness they had before cancer.

your smile, the glint in your eye, or your infectious laugh. Don't deprive someone else of enjoying all that by closing the door on intimacy.

87. During my treatment, I was pretty sick. My husband was a great caregiver. He fed me, helped me dress, and even bathed me sometimes. I feel grateful and loving towards him. But for some reason, our sex life seems to have died down. What's going on?

It sounds like your husband was an invaluable ally during your treatment. You describe him as caring for you in a total way—almost as if you were a loved child. But that could be part of the problem that you are facing now.

Many couples find that once they have shifted into a patient-and-caregiver or parent-and-child mode, it's hard to switch back to another way of connecting. Though they may want to resume a partnership of equals, it can be hard to do after a long period of illness. It's understandable that someone who treated you like a baby may appear more like a parent or nurse than a sexual being. The opposite is equally true—if someone has been ill for a long time, with little energy, perhaps throwing up or soiling the bed linens, that person may seem more like a child or patient than a suitable romantic partner. So, first of all, don't assume that your sexual relationship is over—it has just been in storage for a while. It will take time for both of you to adjust to the new status of your partnership, and to resume your former roles. There are many ways to help this along.

Some couples find that even a brief time away from the place where you were cared for can make a difference. "We had to get away from the scene of the crime," says Lenny, who cared for his wife, Lorna, for nearly a year in their apartment, when she was treated for breast cancer—a treatment that included several setbacks when she developed numerous infections. Lenny and Lorna found that a week in the Bahamas ("Without the kids!" stresses Lenny) made a real difference in getting them connected again.

But even if you can't get away, it can help to start "dating" again. Set aside time for dinner or a movie a couple of times a week. Buy some scented candles for the bedroom—and maybe even some new sheets and pillows which were not part of the sickroom. For some couples, erotic videos can help them to feel sexual again.

But this process should not be rushed. Practice and frequency may increase desire and comfort over time. Start slowly, with kissing and holding. Then you may want to move to slow and sensuous touching. And most of all, don't forget that hands-on caregiving is a rich and wonderful part of a relationship. Congratulate yourselves for the way you got through the cancer experience. And enjoy reconnecting in the time frame that's right for you.

88. The treatment I had affected my ovaries and left me unable to have a child. I'm broken-hearted because all I ever wanted was to be a mother. My friends and family keep telling me that my partner and I can adopt. How do I let them know that I am not interested in that, and that their suggestions are not helpful?

Cancer treatment brings with it many changes, some of which involve loss. In this case, you have suffered the very particular loss of a dream that was deeply meaningful to you. It's important that you grieve this loss as much as possible before you can consider any of the options open to you. You may continue to feel that adoption is of no interest to you, or you may find that that feeling changes over time. It's clearly no one else's business whether you decide to build your family by adopting.

But the question you're asking also involves how to communicate to others that this is not a topic that's open to discussion. It may be that your strong feelings of hurt and anger are getting in the way of your making a simple statement. This is understandable, given the depth of your grief. In addition to being angry about the effects of your treatment on your ability to conceive, you may also feel that the suggestion itself is insensitive, because it doesn't take into account the reality of your loss, and implies that your painful problem can be readily solved. Many people don't know how to offer comfort to someone who is grieving, and do so in a way that seems clumsy or insensitive. It may feel to you as if it's better for them to say nothing at all. But remember—they don't know that. They want to reach out in some way, but aren't sure how. You can let them know that their suggestion isn't helpful to you, or say that this topic is not open for discussion now.

89. My chemo treatments made me infertile and now I am considering adoption. Will I be able to adopt given my cancer history?

Many cancer survivors have adopted children after treatment. In general, your health *is* a concern for agencies, and although there have been rare cases of those with advanced (but stable) illness getting approval, it helps to be considered well. This will require a letter from your oncologist confirming that you are now healthy. The letter should also state how long you have been cancer free and that this is the expectation for many years to come. This means, of course, that if you have just finished treatment, you may need to wait a while before you move forward.

The adoption application process does require health information from adoptive parents, and any questions on this subject should be answered honestly. As long as you have the accompanying documents to further explain your cancer history, you should be fine. As we know, not everyone understands cancer and what it means, so it is possible that the agency staff may be misinformed about the significance of your history; this is where full documentation from your doctor on your health status can be really helpful. Part of the assessment process will probably be a visit to your home; this will be another chance for you to educate the agency about your history and current wellness. We recommend that if this happens you request a social worker or staff person who is familiar with cancer and is therefore more able to understand what it means for your health and the care of the child.

Consulting with a social worker who is an adoption specialist as well as a lawyer is also necessary during the adoption process. There may be different requirements depending on whether you are applying for an international adoption or a domestic one. This is something that fluctuates, and an adoption social worker would be the best resource for up-to-date information.

There are web sites to go to for more information such as BreastCancer.org at http://www.breastcancer.org/adoption.html as well as Fertile Hope Network at www.fertilehope.org.

PART EIGHT

Growth, Change, and Spirituality

When I got my diagnosis I vowed to change—to stop and smell the roses, spend more time with loved ones, and take up yoga and meditation. But so far I haven't done any of these things. Does this mean I'm not a successful survivor?

Since my diagnosis, I kind of feel that God let me down, and I've lost my belief. Will I get it back?

I have the weird feeling that, in a way, my cancer was a good thing—a kind of wake-up call that told me I was living too fast, and not enjoying simple, everyday pleasures. Is this a strange way to look an event that everyone dreads?

More . . .

90. I view my cancer as a wake-up call, telling me that I had lost sight of what's meaningful in life. When I got my diagnosis I vowed to change—to stop and smell the roses, spend more time with loved ones, and take up yoga and meditation. But so far I haven't done any of these things. Does this mean I'm not a successful survivor?

First of all, there is no one definition of a successful survivor. There are as many different ways of succeeding as there are survivors. And no matter what goals you may set for yourself, getting there is a process, not a one-time event. None of us can change old habits overnight, and you shouldn't expect yourself to do so. But the first question is: Do you really want to make the changes you talk about? Do they come from deep inside you, or are they suggestions made by people you know, or an article you've read? Perhaps someone has implied that if you *don't* make these changes, you cannot be happy—or perhaps more importantly, healthy. Start by taking off the pressure and reflecting on whether the activities you mention are truly meaningful to you. If they are, then by all means, keep them in sight. But start small. Maybe you can add one activity at a time. And not everything requires special classes, or a lot of time and money. Perhaps you could begin by simply slowing your pace a little. One woman told us that she walked through the city park for years, passing many statues. After her cancer experience, she slowed her pace, and strolled. For the first time, she read all the names on the statues and knew who they were! This was a revelation to her after years of not really "seeing" them.

If you continue to feel that you want to learn new things like yoga or meditation, there may be places in your community where you can do that. Sometimes cancer organizations or groups offer such classes—as do community groups like

YMCAs or YWCAs. You can also find such instruction on CDs and DVDs.

But no matter what changes you decide to make, try not to constantly measure your progress, in the way an eager dieter keeps jumping on the scale. It's better to move at your own pace, and then, many months or a year down the line, look at how your life has changed, bit by bit, over time.

Dave comments:

My diagnosis was a wake-up call. First, it made me realize that I had made a grave mistake by putting off my screening until my cancers were in advanced stages. I quickly began to realize that I was going to be just as responsible for the success of my treatments.

My instincts drove me to pester my family and friends to schedule their medical screenings, appointing myself as the "poster boy" for the price paid for putting off screening.

As time passed, through my surgery and treatment experiences, and now, in my post-treatment life, I have become active on several fronts to help develop programs for cancer survivors. Not everyone can become involved in this manner. One survivor I know says he would not waste his time with these programs; he would rather be involved with activities that he enjoys, such as ballroom dancing. I think that is a great answer to post treatment. The important point is to realize that life is now, and that doing things that you are driven to do is the right answer, no matter what those things are.

*Religious
or spiritual
feelings may
be reevaluated
after cancer;
this can be
healthy.*

91. Before I got cancer, religion was a large part of my life. I went to church regularly, and had a strong faith. But since my diagnosis, I kind of feel that God let me down, and I've lost my belief. Will I get it back?

Many survivors struggle with these feelings of disillusionment with a faith that may have been meaningful until cancer entered the picture. One group member wept as she reported approaching her church and finding the door locked. She said, "I knew the side door was open—it always is. But I felt so angry that I didn't even try it. That locked door just seemed to say it all—I felt shut out from all the support and help I got before." A Jewish woman said, "I used to be so observant. I lit candles every Friday night and went to synagogue on every holiday. I thought I was a good person, and a good Jew. So why did I get sick? It makes me mad, and I feel like I don't have any belief left."

For a response to this issue, let's turn to Jane Mather, Director of Chaplaincy Services at Memorial Sloan-Kettering Cancer Center. She says, "It's important to remember that being angry at God isn't a sign of a lack of faith—it's a part of an ongoing relationship. As in a marriage, a relationship can grow from fighting. You may be able to deepen your relationship if you accept your anger, and engage in a dialog with God about your feelings."

"If someone found religion important before their cancer, they may need to figure out how much of that faith they want to pick up, how much of it is still applicable for them. How we take care of our bodies changes, so how we take care of our spirit has to change, too. It's important to ask, 'What do I need now?'"

In this vein, a number of survivors also say their faith is revitalized by the challenge of cancer—or talk about finding faith for the first time. This faith may come in many forms. One woman spoke of having a severe infection while on treatment for ovarian cancer. She described lying in the intensive care unit late at night, and feeling very alone. "Suddenly," she said "it all changed. I suddenly felt this sense of community with all the people who had ever felt alone, who had ever suffered. My mind just kept thinking of all the things that humanity has gone through for thousands of years. I felt a kind of oneness with the world that gave me peace."

The process of reevaluation that accompanies a cancer experience can bring with it multiple losses, but also many gains—including in the spiritual realm. Mather reminds us: "Throwing it all out and starting again can be good!"

92. Before I got cancer, I thought it was the worst thing that could happen to anyone. And believe me, treatment was no picnic. But now I have the weird feeling that, in a way, my cancer was a good thing—a kind of wake-up call that told me I was living too fast, and not enjoying simple, everyday pleasures. I've also met some great new friends, like a guy at work who told me he had the same disease and the great people in my support group. Is this a strange way to look an event that everyone dreads?

No! For every survivor who does characterize cancer as "the worst thing that has ever happened to me," there is someone like you, who sees the experience differently. Anything that changes us, tests us, or challenges us can lead to growth that might not have taken place otherwise. Would you have become friendly with your colleague at work if you hadn't shared a powerful experience? You certainly wouldn't have joined a group where you learned how much mutual support human beings can offer to others. You may also, as many survivors do, make positive changes in your life—making time for family, friends, and other things that are important to you—a step you might not have taken if illness hadn't entered your life. Some survivors say that their feelings about themselves change after treatment. One woman observed "I never thought of myself as a particularly strong person. But during my treatment I learned how strong I really am." Another survivor reflected "During chemo I had to reach down inside myself and pull out all the faith and hope that was in there. There was more than I thought!"

Cancer can be life-changing in many positive ways.

These observations don't mean that cancer is a good experience. But they do mean that good things can come out of it, if one is open to them. Some people don't feel open to them right away; one young man in a support group said, "If cancer is a gift, show me to the returns counter!" But others will feel as you do—that the complex experience of having cancer has added a valuable dimension to their lives.

Judy comments:

I was always worried about getting cancer, or that people I loved would get cancer. But then, I worried about everything. I was worried that the subway would stop underground and that a deranged person would shoot everyone, so I took slow busses instead. I was worried that the plane would crash, so I traveled seldom, with great trepidation, and only for short flights. And so on. But over time, as I've been surviving lung cancer for four and a half years, I feel much more relaxed about everything. I've stopped waiting for something terrible to happen, because I realize that worrying about terrible things doesn't prevent them from happening. I've switched from an anxious, "warding off" mentality to a coping mentality. I finally believe that I can't control major events, but that I can cope with them, have courage in the face of them, and make significant choices no matter what happens. What a relief! And now I take the subway anywhere, and have traveled to Europe three times in a year and a half. Yet I have cancer all the time.

I feel less scared of death. I think of it as an inevitable part of life, rather than as a unique catastrophe. This fact makes me want to live as well as possible, and makes me value the life I have more than ever. Since my diagnosis I've carved out a life that I love and enjoy. I work only part time, when before I worked all the time, and I have re-invented myself professionally. I am involved in several reading seminars: two are based around reading fiction, (a long love of mine), and two are based on psychotherapy cases and professional readings with colleagues. I love photography, and enjoy my digital camera: recently I've been making greeting cards out of my photographs. I learned to meditate, and I meet with my meditation group regularly. One of the teachings of meditation is the value of being fully in each moment. I value my relationships with my husband and daughter more and more deeply, and I accept them much more uncritically than I ever did. In turn, they're more and more close, trusting, loving, and warm with me.

So the truth is, I love my life the way it is now, and I hope I would love it just as much if I didn't have metastatic lung cancer anymore. It's not all great all the time, though, and when I don't feel so well or when I have a setback medically I can get mournful and angry about my illness. A key point for me is that I have felt relatively well all this time. If I were in constant pain, or nauseated, or disfigured or immobilized, I cannot be confident that I'd feel as positively as I do about the cancer experience.

93. I finished chemo last month. Cancer treatment was so tough, I would love to help others get through it by donating my time to a cancer organization or hospital. Where is the best place for me to volunteer?

It's terrific that you want to help others with cancer. And there's no question that you would have a lot to offer them, after all you've been through and all you've learned. As for finding someplace to volunteer, there are probably a wealth of places in your area—the local chapter of the American

Cancer Society, hospitals, friendly visitor programs, and others. But you may want to hold off for a little while. You've just finished your own treatment, and are only beginning the process of digesting what you've been through. You may not even know yet all the ways that cancer has affected you. You owe it to yourself to take your own journey for a while, before giving your time and energy to others.

It could also be that being around people undergoing treatment for cancer could be more upsetting than you think. Memories of your own treatment may surface, bringing back feelings of distress or even illness. Once you have a little distance from your own experience, this could be easier.

And finally, is it possible that your wish to help others is a way of avoiding your own process of reflection and processing? This doesn't mean that your impulse to reach out isn't sincere or heartfelt—only that you may need to do a little healing before giving all you have to offer.

94. My hospital offers classes for survivors. There is one in collage, and another in writing. I'd like to try them, but have no artistic talent. Should I bother?

Of course! Since these classes are being offered by your hospital, chances are they are not about "talent" or producing a finished product, but rather about expressing your feelings about your illness in a variety of ways. Many survivors tell us that art, writing, or photography classes are very meaningful to them, even if they had no interest in these activities before. Sometimes the powerful feelings brought about by a cancer experience are actually hard to talk about. It may be easier to describe them in another way. And even if talking about your experience comes more readily to you, working in another medium can deepen your understand of the impact that your illness has had on you. Sometimes you can also connect with others in the class in a way that is more relaxed than an "official" group setting.

On the last night of one of our eight-week groups for women who had completed treatment, we suggested that instead of talking, the participants make collages, using pictures that spoke to their cancer experience. In the group there was a woman named Joyce, whose thick brown hair reached past her ears, looking as if it had grown back completely following her treatment. As the group worked on their collages, she busily cut out and pasted many images of women with long, flowing hair. Another member said "Oh—I get it, that's all about losing your hair." Joyce replied "Yes, it was especially hard for me, because, before chemo, I could sit on my hair." There was silence in the room as everyone realized how profoundly cancer had affected Joyce's image of herself. Whereas hair loss had been hard for all who experienced it, it had radically changed the way Joyce looked and felt. In the eight weeks of group discussion, she had never mentioned this fact; only by using pictures could she describe what she had lost—to the group, and to herself.

PART NINE

Cancer as a Chronic Illness

I have metastatic disease. Am I still a survivor?

When I recovered from my cancer, everyone treated me like a hero because I "beat it." Now I'm sick again, and feel that I've let everyone, including my doctor, down. Is this normal?

I have metastatic prostate cancer. My wife says that I should stop working, because the stress might tire me out too much. Sometimes I even forget I'm sick. Who's right?

More . . .

*Many people
survive with
cancer, rather
than beyond it.*

95. I have metastatic disease. Am I still a survivor?

This question doesn't have a simple answer, because it depends very much on whom you ask. The National Cancer Institute has long used the following definition, which certainly includes those who require treatment once again.

"An individual is considered a cancer survivor from the time of diagnosis, through the balance of his or her life. Family members, friends, and caregivers are also impacted by the survivorship experience and are therefore included in this definition."

Many of those who have had cancer find this a meaningful way to view their experience, while others disagree. Roz Kleban, LCSW, who for many years has conducted groups for those with metastatic breast cancer, says that many members of this group resent being called survivors. "To them, the term survivor means 'finished.' These women feel that they will never be finished with treatment."

On the other hand, a number of members of another group for those with advanced disease feel that the word does apply to them, even though their cancer situation is ongoing. Let's listen to Judy, who is part of this remarkable and spirited group.

Judy comments:

I think the term "survivor" can mean different things in different cases. I guess I would say I'm a survivor with ongoing disease. Everyday I survive cancer, I'm a survivor. But there is a difference between me and someone who has been disease-free for, say, six years. With metastatic lung cancer, I don't expect to be cured. So I don't expect to be a survivor in the sense of having outlived my cancer and put it behind me. I live on a daily basis with my cancer;

we coexist. My hope is to survive with it for as long as possible, and to have as good a quality of life as possible. I'm proud of how well I've survived for the past four and a half years, and I'm glad every day that I've survived again. Of course, if in the meantime something comes up which does "cure" the cancer, that would be great. And then I would be a different sort of survivor.

96. When I recovered from my cancer, everyone treated me like a hero because I "beat it." Now I'm sick again, and feel that I've let everyone, including my doctor, down. Is this normal?

The answer to your question may be contained in the question itself. In our society, and especially in the media, cancer is often depicted as a kind of intense and grueling sporting event. Making it through treatment is frequently referred to as "beating" the disease. But this is really not a fair analogy. Although it takes toughness to get through treatment for cancer, it is not toughness that beats the cancer—it is treatment, which either works or does not. It's great for people to feel that their resiliency played a role in their recovery, but this isn't the same as saying that their resiliency—on its own—brought it about, or that it can keep them free of disease.

We are delighted to see that, over the last twenty years, patients have grown increasingly empowered, and feel more than ever that they are vital and active members of their health care team. We would never want them to lose the belief that they, their proactive choices, and their fighting spirit all matter. But we are also distressed that the flipside of this sense of power is a feeling of being totally responsible for the success or failure of their treatment. You, your attitude, and your personal strength are only part of the reasons for recovery.

Cancer is a complex disease. We don't know why a treatment that cures one person may not completely eradicate disease in another. Until we know more, it is too simplistic to say that a person's attitude or thoughts were not tough enough to keep disease at bay.

Finally, try not to be too preoccupied by the thoughts and feelings of those around you. We would bet that your friends, family, and doctor all know how hard you have worked to get well, and are only sorry that you must face treatment again.

97. I have metastatic prostate cancer, and I know that my medical situation is quite serious, even though the medication I'm on now is keeping my disease pretty stable. My wife says that I should stop working, because the stress might tire me out too much. But getting to the office, staying in touch, and giving the younger folks guidance and advice makes me feel good. Sometimes I even forget I'm sick. Who's right?

It would be hard to call your wife wrong, when what she wants is for you to stay healthy. But it sounds like in this case, she isn't making the right call for you and you might need to make this decision for yourself.

More and more, the medical profession is beginning to view cancer as a chronic illness. This means that, like a diabetic, you may always need to be on treatment. But it also means that you can go about your life, including work, as long as you feel that's what you want to do. Recently, a woman with ovarian cancer, who for many years had been taking part in our meetings for those with metastatic illness, left the group—not because she was too sick to continue, but because she accepted a job. It had been important to Sylvia to acknowledge her illness, to discuss it with others, and to learn what she could from her fellow group members. But it was also important to her to feel useful and active, which prompted her to shift her focus away from the world of cancer.

The point here is that you have options. If you need to stop working, because you're not up to the same level of energy, then that may be the right choice for you. If you *want* to stop in order to spend more time with your children or grandchildren, or to travel to certain places while you are well enough to do so, then that might your best option. But you don't *have* to stop working simply because you have a certain diagnosis. Doing so would be treating yourself more like a statistic than a real person—which is what you are, sick or well.

98. I have advanced lung cancer, which I have been living with for three years. During that time, my doctor has tried eight chemotherapies to treat my disease. Now she says that my most recent treatment didn't work, and that the options that remain are real long shots, and unlikely to control my disease. I'm tired of being on chemo, dealing with side effects, and being tired much of the time. I'd like to say 'no thanks' to further treatment. Am I a quitter?

It's pretty clear from what you have said that you are far from a quitter. Most people find chemotherapy challenging, even if they go through it only once. In your case, you have done it eight times; this shows how determined you have been to overcome your disease and get well. But only you can decide when and whether to stop treatment. Many people tell us that this is a hard and lonely decision-making process. Sometimes they experience pressure from family, or

Even when a cure is not being offered, there is still medical help available to you.

even their health care team, to "try everything." But again, as much as you may want to respond to the wishes of others, this choice is yours and yours alone. (Which is, of course, the good news as well as the hard news.)

It sounds like you have had a frank discussion with your doctor about what your treatment options are at this point. This is, of course, an important component in making your choice about how to proceed. Some people also choose to speak to a religious advisor, counselor, or social worker to sort through their thoughts. But no matter who you choose to speak with , you are the ultimate arbiter of what is right for you.

99. Is there any help for me if treatment isn't an option?

Palliative care

Medical care, the goal of which is to relieve pain and discomfort, rather than to cure a disease or condition.

Hospice care

Medical, psychosocial, and spiritual care given to medically ill people when they have ceased to seek curative treatment; often given in patient's own home under the auspices of a specialized facility.

Yes. Perhaps you have heard the term **palliative care** or **hospice care**. These are terms that are often misunderstood to mean care that is given only at the end of life. Many people mistakenly believe that if they accept this kind of care, they will die shortly thereafter. Some think it means they will get no treatment at all. This is not the case. In most cases, people who die of an illness have had it for a number of years (as you have). Palliative care can actually enhance quality of life during that time. Any symptoms you have *will* be treated. The goal of such care is to allow you to be free of pain or discomfort in a way that allows you to interact maximally with friends and family, and enjoy the pleasures of life without the rigors of harsh or debilitating treatments.

Palliative care may be offered in a number of places. Some hospitals provide such care. There are also facilities dedicated to this type of care. They usually differ greatly from hospitals, and are peaceful, quiet, attractive, and welcoming. A third option is to receive care at home. This is what many people choose to do. It enables them to be in familiar and comfortable surroundings, do many of the things they enjoy, and be with friends (and even cats and dogs.)

Be aware that deciding to discontinue curative chemotherapy does not mean you will not be cared for. The movement to offer patients palliative care is growing continually, as the medical profession (and patients themselves) recognize the humane (and very human) care that it provides.

100. Where can I get more information on survivorship?

The Appendix on the next few pages offers a wide variety of resources on survivorship and other cancer-related topics.

Appendix

Organizations
General Cancer and Survivorship Information and Support

American Cancer Society (ACS)
800-ACS-2345 (800-227-2345)
www.cancer.org
Organization that offers a variety of services to patients and families. The ACS also supports research, provides materials, and conducts educational programs.

Cancer*Care*, Inc.
800-813-HOPE (800-813-4673)
www.cancercare.org
National nonprofit agency that offers free support, information, financial assistance, and practical help to patients and survivors; services available in person, over the phone, and through the Web site.

A Cancer Survivor's Compendium
www.hopeandhealing.com
Directory of resources for living well after cancer.

Cancer Survivors Project
www.cancersurvivorsproject.org
Community resource for long-term survivors of cancer.

Cancervive
800-486-2873
www.cancervive.org
Offers support groups, educational materials, and practical information to patients and survivors.

Gilda's Club

http://www.gildasclub.org/WhereToFindUs/FindUs/tabid/115/Default.aspx

Organization with multiple locations around the country offering support and activities for cancer patients.

Lance Armstrong Foundation

512-236-8820

www.livestrong.org

Helps patients and survivors with advocacy, education, public health and research, as well as the **LIVESTRONG** Resource for Cancer Survivors.

National Cancer Institute (NCI)

800-4-CANCER (800-422-6237)

www.cancer.gov

bethesdatrials.cancer.gov

Comprehensive site offering all types of information about cancer, prevention, definitions, clinical trial information, recipes, and links to cancer centers.

National Coalition for Cancer Survivorship

877-622-7937

www.canceradvocacy.org

Support to cancer survivors and their loved ones; provides information and resources on support, advocacy and quality-of-life issues.

OncoLink

www.oncolink.com

Resources for patients, families and health care workers that is written by health professionals, as well as survivors.

People Living With Cancer

703-299-0150

www.plwc.org

Patient information web site of the American Society of Clinical Oncologists.

Post-Treatment Resource Program of Memorial Sloan-Kettering Cancer Center
212-717-3527
http://www.mskcc.org/mskcc/html/19409.cfm
Offers psychosocial support and guidance to cancer survivors and family members.

The Wellness Community
888-793-WELL (888-793-9355)
www.thewellnesscommunity.org
Provides free psychosocial support to cancer patients and their families; offers groups on stress reduction and cancer education workshops, nutrition guidance, exercise sessions, and social events.

Legal and Workplace Issues

Cancer Legal Resource Center
213-THE-CLRC (743-2572)
http://www.disabilityrightslegalcenter.org/about/cancerlegalresource.cfm
Provides information on cancer-related legal issues for patients and survivors.

Cancer and Careers
www.cancerandcareers.org
Provides a free workbook, educational resources, support and information for cancer patients and survivors, as well as their employers; focus is on working through treatment and returning to work.

Young Adults

Fertile Hope
888-994-4673
www.fertilehope.org
Nonprofit organization dedicated to helping cancer survivors with fertility issues.

Healthy Young Attitude
www.hya.org
Network of young adults whose lives have been affected by cancer.

I'm Too Young for This!

www.imtooyoungforthis.org

A Web site for discussion of the cancer experience.

Let's Connect

www.letsconnect.org

Web site designed to connect young adults who have experienced serious illness. Resources, camps, and scholarship information are also available.

National Collegiate Cancer Foundation

www.collegiatecancer.org

Services and support for college students who are cancer survivors.

Planet Cancer

www.planetcancer.org

Web site for young adults with cancer; playful and fun approach.

Prepare to Live (P2L)

www.preparetolive.org

Non-profit organization founded and managed by cancer survivors, offering information and support to young adults with cancer.

Steps for Living

877-735-4673

www.stepsforliving.org

Non-profit support and advocacy agency for adolescents and young adults with cancer; emphasis is on quality of life and psychosocial support.

Surviving and Moving Forward (the SAMFund)

www.thesamfund.org

Non-profit organization created to assist young adult survivors of cancer between the ages of 17 and 30 with their transition to post-treatment phase; offers financial support through the distribution of grants and scholarships.

Ulman Cancer Fund for Young Adults
888-393-FUND (3863)
www.ulmanfund.org
Provides support programs, education and resources to young
adult survivors, as well as their families and friends.

Young Adults with Cancer
800-GRP-ROOM (800-477-7666)
www.youngadultswithcancer.org
Young Adult Cancer Awareness program.

Women

Mautner Project: The National Lesbian Health Organization
http://www.mautnerproject.org/health_information/Cancer/
Provides support and information for lesbian, bisexual, and
transgender women with cancer, and their families.

Team Survivor
www.teamsurvivor.org
Provides exercise and health education programs free-of-charge
for women with a past or present diagnosis of cancer.

National Asian Women's Health Organization (NAWHO)
415-989-9747
www.nawho.org
Dedicated to improving health status of Asian women and their
families through research, education, and public policy programs;
resources in English, Cantonese, Laotian, Vietnamese and
Korean.

Childhood Cancer Survivors

Beyond the Cure
314-241-1600
www.BeyondTheCure.org
Organization for survivors of childhood cancer, offering
information about late effects of treatment.

Outlook: Life Beyond Childhood Cancer
www.outlook-life.org
Web site offering information on health issues and financial
issues, as well as other resources.

The Stephen T. Marchello Scholarship Foundation
www.stmfoundation.org
Organization allocating post secondary scholarship monies to
survivors of childhood cancer.

Complementary Therapies

About Herbs, Botanicals & Other Products
http://www.mskcc.org/mskcc/html/11570.cfm
Web site led by an oncology-trained pharmacist that provides
information about herbs and other products, including a clinical
summary for each agent and details about adverse side effects,
interactions and potential benefits or problems.

Center for Mind-Body Medicine
202-966-7338
www.cmbm.org
Addresses the mental, emotional, social, physical and spiritual
sides of health and illness.

**National Center for Complementary and Alternative Medicine
(NCCAM)**
888-644-6226
www.nccam.nih.gov
Provides information on research, events and clinical trials in
complementary medicine.

Hospice & Palliative Care

Center to Advance Palliative Care (CAPC)
www.getpalliativecare.org
Information for patients and families, including description of
palliative care, and provider directory.

Hospice Education Institute

800-331-1620

www.hospiceworld.org

Helps patients and their families find hospice and palliative care services in their communities.

National Association for Home Care

202-547-7424

www.nahc.org

Provides information on choosing hospice and home care providers.

National Hospice and Palliative Care Organization (NHPCO)

800-658-8898

www.caringinfo.org

An association of programs that provide hospice and palliative care.

Patient Advocacy

Patient Advocate Foundation (PAF)

800-532-5274

www.patientadvocate.org

Provides education, legal and insurance information, and referrals to cancer patients and survivors.

Survivorship Clinics

Abramson Cancer Center of the University of Pennsylvania

800-789-7366

www.penncancer.org

Dana-Farber Cancer Institute

617-632-5100

www.dana-farber.org/pat/surviving/adult-onset/default.html

Fred Hutchinson Cancer Research Center

206-667-2814

www.fhcrc.org/patient/support/survivorship

Memorial Sloan-Kettering Cancer Center

212-639-2581

www.mskcc.org/mskcc/html/64918.cfm

147

Ohio State University Comprehensive Cancer Center
800-293-5066
www.jamesline.com

UCLA's Jonsson Comprehensive Cancer Center
310-206-1404
www.cancer.mednet.ucla.edu

University of Colorado Cancer Center
303-239-3397
www.uccc.info

Bladder Cancer

Bladder Cancer Webcafé
www.blcwebcafe.org
Offers information on latest in bladder cancer treatments, clinical trials and
alternatives, as well as support.

Breast Cancer

Living Beyond Breast Cancer
610-645-4567
800-753-5222 (toll-free helpline)
www.lbbc.org
Provides educational materials, a quarterly newsletter, a Young Survivors
Network, and a toll-free helpline at 800-753-5222.

Pink-Link
310-995-5204
www.pink-link.org
Online searchable database of women affected by breast cancer, as well as friends
and co-survivors.

SHARE: Self-help for Women with Breast or Ovarian Cancer
866-891-2392
www.sharecancersupport.org
Provides free support groups, educational forums, wellness programs, events,
newsletter, and toll-free hotline.

Sisters Network, Inc.
866-781-1808
www.sistersnetworkinc.org
Seeks to increase local and national attention to the impact of breast cancer in the African-American community; all chapters run by breast cancer survivors.

Susan G. Komen Breast Cancer Foundation
Helpline: 1-800-IMAWARE
www.komen.org
Provides support for those with breast cancer and advocacy for a cure.

Young Survival Coalition
877-972-1011
www.youngsurvival.org
International network of breast cancer survivors and supporters dedicated to the concerns of breast cancer patients and survivors younger than 40 years old.

Colorectal Cancer

Colon Cancer Alliance
877-422-2030
www.ccalliance.org
Offers patient support, as well as resources, news on research, and advocacy.

United Ostomy Association, Inc.
800-826-0826 (6:30am to 4:30pm, PST)
www.uoa.org
Helps ostomy patients through mutual support; provides information and sends volunteers to visit new ostomy patients.

Esophageal Cancer

Esophageal Cancer Awareness Association
866-730-ECAA (866-730-3222)
607-257-1141 (local)
www.ECaware.org
Organization providing support for esophageal cancer patients and caregivers.

Gynecological Cancers

Gynecologic Cancer Foundation
www.thegcf.org
Encourages public awareness of prevention, early diagnosis and proper treatment as well as supporting research and training related to gynecologic cancers.

National Ovarian Cancer Coalition (NOCC)
888-OVARIAN (888-682-7426)
www.ovarian.org
Raises awareness about ovarian cancer; promotes education and offers support.

Ovarian Cancer National Alliance (OCNA)
202-331-1332
www.ovariancancer.org
Works to increase understanding of ovarian cancer and to advocate for research; distributes materials and sponsors an annual advocacy conference for survivors and families.

SHARE: Self-help for Women with Breast or Ovarian Cancer
866-891-2392
www.sharecancersupport.org
Provides free support groups, educational forums, wellness programs, events, newsletter, and toll-free hotline.

Vulva Awareness Cancer Organization
www.vaco.co.uk
carolvaco2003@yahoo.co.uk
Provides a community listserv, educational resources, support and assistance for women who have been through vulval cancer.

Head and Neck Cancer

Support for People With Oral and Head and Neck Cancer
800-377-0928
www.spohnc.org
Provides education, support, a "Survivor to Survivor" network, information on clinical trials and a newsletter.

Kidney Cancer

Kidney Cancer Association
800-850-9132
www.kidneycancerassociation.org
Supports research and offers printed materials about the diagnosis and treatment of kidney cancer, as well as providing support and a physician referral information.

Lung Cancer

Lung Cancer Alliance
800-298-2436
www.lungcanceralliance.org
Offers programs to help improve the quality of life of people with lung cancer and their families.

Hematologic Cancers

The Leukemia and Lymphoma Society
800-955-4572
www.lls.org
Voluntary health organization dedicated to funding blood cancer research and providing education and patient services to improve quality of life.

Michael A. Hunter Memorial Scholarship Award
http://www.oc-cf.org/default.asp?contentID=627
Awards annual scholarships to help improve the quality of life for those affected by leukemia.

Prostate Cancer

American Foundation for Urologic Disease (AFUD)
800-242-2383
www.afud.org
Provides information on urologic disease and dysfunctions, including prostate cancer; offers prostate cancer support groups.

Malecare Prostate Cancer Support

212-844-8369

www.malecare.com

Non-profit organization providing a multilingual website; also in-person and online support groups, including a special group and articles specific for gay men with prostate cancer.

UsTOO International, Inc.

800-80-US TOO (800-808-7866)

www.ustoo.org

Prostate cancer support organization; goals are to educate men newly diagnosed with prostate cancer, offer support groups, and provide the latest information about treatment for this disease.

Sarcoma

Sarcoma Awareness Foundation

407-884-9670

www.sarcomaawareness.com

Goal is to promote awareness of sarcoma, as well as to raise funding for research to help find a cure.

Sarcoma Foundation of America

301-520-7648

www.curesarcoma.org

Dedicated to raising funds for sarcoma research, patient networking and support.

Thyroid Cancer

ThyCa: Thyroid Cancer Survivors' Association

877-588-7904

www.thyca.org

Provides support and education for thyroid cancer survivors and their families.

Fatigue

Association of Cancer Online Resources (ACOR)

www.acor.org (Click on "Mailing Lists," then on "CANCER-FATIGUE.")

Online discussion site dedicated to cancer- and treatment-related fatigue.

National Cancer Institute/PDQ Fatigue
www.cancer.gov (enter "fatigue" in search slot)
Part of the NCI's comprehensive cancer information site.

Pain

American Alliance of Cancer Pain Initiatives
608-265-4013
www.aacpi.wisc.edu
Provides advocacy for state and regional pain initiatives.

American Pain Foundation
888-615-7246
www.painfoundation.org
Offers Pain Action Guide and other informational material, as well as support
and advocacy.

Partners Against Pain
www.partnersagainstpain.com
Includes news updates, pain control guides, support groups, resources and
information.

Books and Other Publications

Pamphlet
Facing Forward Series: Life After Cancer Treatment
The National Cancer Institute

Books
Feuerstein, M, PhD, MPH and Findley, P, DrPH, SW.
The Cancer Survivor's Guide: The Essential Handbook to Life After Cancer.
New York, Marlowe & Company, 2006.

Hewitt M, Ganz P, eds. *From Cancer Patient to Cancer Survivor: Lost in
Transition.* Washington, D.C., National Academies Press, 2006.

Holland, J, MD and Lewis, S. *The Human Side of Cancer.* New York, Harper
Collins, 2001.

Ganz, P (ed.). *Cancer Survivorship-Today and Tomorrow.* New York, Springer
Publishing, 2007.

Glossary

A

ADA (the Americans With Disabilities Act): Legislation passed in 1991 to ensure that people with health problems—or a history of them—do not suffer discrimination in the workplace or elsewhere.

Addictive: Word describing something that is physically or psychologically habit-forming, so that discontinuation causes extreme distress or discomfort.

Antidepressant medication: Drugs used to alleviate the symptoms of clinical depression, such as sadness, insomnia, and lack of energy.

B

Bone marrow transplant, allogeneic: A medical procedure in which healthy **stem cells** are donated by another person (a donor), who may or may not be related to the patient, but whose cells must be a good genetic match, and given to the patient after high-dose chemotherapy; sometimes used as part of the treatment for cancers that are in the bone marrow, such as leukemia and multiple myeloma.

Bone marrow transplant, autologous: A medical procedure in which cells are obtained from one's own bone marrow, frozen, and reinfused after high-dose chemotherapy is given.

C

Chemo brain: A term coined by cancer survivors to describe problems with memory loss and concentration following chemotherapy treatment.

Chemotherapy: The use of drugs to treat cancer throughout the body.

COBRA (Consolidated Omnibus Budget Reconciliation Act): Law passed by congress in 1986 providing continuation of group health coverage that might otherwise be terminated.

D

Denial: An emotional state that permits a person to keep painful facts out of consciousness in order to avoid the pain of acknowledging them.

Depression, clinical: An emotional disorder characterized by feelings of sadness, loss of appetite, insomnia, and inability to concentrate, often involving changes in brain chemistry.

Dopamine: A neurotransmitter in the central nervous system that regulates emotion and movement.

E

Essential functions of job: Legal term referring to those aspects of a job that are integral to performance of the job.

F

FMLA (Family and Medical Leave Act): Law passed by congress in 1993 stating that in most cases employers must grant an employee up to 12 work weeks of unpaid leave during any 12-month period, in order to care for an immediate family member, or because of their own serious health condition.

H

Hormonal treatment: Treatment that blocks the effect of hormones in hormone-dependent cancers.

Hospice care: Medical, psychosocial, and spiritual care given to medically ill people when they have ceased to seek curative treatment; often given in patient's own home under the auspices of a specialized facility.

Hypochondriac: A person who worries excessively about being or becoming ill, often with no foundation.

L

Late effects: Effects of cancer treatment on one's health, which may not appear until years after treatment is given.

M

Mammogram: A low-dose x-ray used to examine the breast, which aids in detecting disease.

Mesothelioma: A rare form of cancer, usually caused by exposure to asbestos.

N

Neurotransmitters: Chemicals made by brain cells to help "communicate" with another cell.

Norepinephrine: A neurotransmitter in the central nervous system, connected with the "fight or flight" response, as well as reaction to stress.

P

Palliative care: Medical care, the goal of which is to relieve pain and discomfort, rather than to cure a disease or condition.

Peripheral neuropathy: Nerve damage in the extremities that may cause numbness, tingling or weakness.

Post-Traumatic Stress Disorder (PTSD): Psychiatric term describing the psychological aftereffects of very stressful or frightening events. Its symptoms may include irritability, memory loss, insomnia, anxiety, or depression.

Post-treatment fatigue: Marked lack of energy or stamina following treatment for cancer; this may be radiation, chemotherapy, or both.

Preexisting conditions: Term used in the insurance industry to describe medical conditions that existed prior to your being covered by a particular carrier.

PSA blood test: Prostate-Specific Antigen test, administered to men to measure the level of a tumor marker for prostate cancer in the blood.

Psychomotor retardation: Slowing down of movement and thinking, often found in those with clinical depression.

Psychotherapy groups: A form of therapy in which patients are treated for emotional problems in a group led by a mental health professional.

R

Radiation therapy: Use of x-rays to shrink tumors and kill cancerous cells.

Reasonable accommodation: Legal term referring to the special allowances, structures, or schedules that a workplace must make to a disabled worker.

S

Sarcoma: A general class of uncommon cancers affecting the connective tissue of the body.

Serotonin: A neurotransmitter created in the central nervous system, often associated with feelings of well-being.

Stem cells: Cells found in most organisms that have the ability to renew themselves, and to become a variety of different types of cells.

Support group: A meeting, which may or may not be led by a professional facilitator, which brings together people with similar struggles to share their experiences.

T

Teaching hospital: Medical facility that not only provides primary medical care, but also offers experimental or unique treatments and conducts research.

Therapist: A professional, often a social worker, psychologist or psychiatrist, who assists people who are in emotional distress.

U

Undue hardship: A legal term referring to loss or damage suffered by a person or company as a result of providing accommodations that they cannot afford.

Index

A

About Herbs, Botanicals & Other Products, 99

Aches and pains, reactions to, 25–26

ADA (Americans With Disabilities Act), 64–65, 67, 82

Addictive, definition of, 15

Admiration from others, reaction to, 51–52

Adoption
 cancer history and, 120–121
 reluctance to consider, 119–120

After-effects
 disclosure to prospective employer, 69
 fatigue as, 56–58, 82, 98–99
 friends' response to, 56–58

Allogeneic bone marrow transplant, definition of, 10

Alprostadil, 112

Americans With Disabilities Act (ADA), 64–65, 67, 82

Antidepressant medication
 definition of, 15
 fear of dependence on, 15–16
 use of, 14–15, 102

Anxiety
 generalization to everyday life, 24–25
 over aches and pains, 25–26
 over follow-up and tests, 26–27, 32–33
 over symptoms (hypochondria), 34–35

Appearance
compliments about, 13–14
 worry over, 110–111, 117–118

Art, expression of feelings in, 130–131

Autologous bone marrow transplant, definition of, 10

B

Baby showers, reaction to, 90–91

Bills, 75–76

Blaming patient, 58–59

Bone marrow transplant
 allogeneic, definition of, 10
 autologous, definition of, 10
 reflection on experience, 10

Bravery
 comparison of self with others, 9
 reaction to admiration for, 51–52

Breast cancer
exercise and, 28
 follow-up in, 31
 hormonal treatment for, 11
 shielding survivor from family member's findings, 61

C

Cancer. *See also specific entries*
 cause of
 blaming patient for, 58–59
 others' inquiries about, 41–43
 patient's quest for, 27–28
 celebrities with, reaction to, 33–34
 as chronic illness, 133–139
 as identity-altering experience, 3–4
 positive changes with, 127–129
 second, 104
 as "wake-up call," 124–125, 127–129

Cancer Information Service, 103

"Case of one," 33–34

Celebrities with cancer, reaction to, 33–34

Chemo brain, 101–102
Chemotherapy
    declining further, 137–139
    definition of, 4
    end of, mixed feelings about, 4–6
    late effects of, 103–104
Childhood history of cancer, 86
Children
    change in relationship with, 62
    communication with, 48–49
    expectations/insensitivity of, 50–51
    younger, later explanation to, 55–56
Chronic illness, cancer as, 133–139
Classes for survivors, 130–131
Clinical depression. *See also* Depression
    definition of, 14
COBRA coverage, 77
College, interruption in, 87–88
Comparable position at work, 65
Compliments
    about appearance, 13–14
    about bravery, 51–52
Concentration, loss of, 101–102
Consolidated Omnibus Reconciliation
    Act (COBRA), 77
Counseling, 34
Creditors, 75–76
Crying, 7–8, 14

D

Dating concerns
    disclosure of cancer history, 107–110
    fear of rejection, 109–110
    worry over appearance, 110–111
Debt, 75–76
Democratic disease, cancer as, 33–34
Denial
    definition of, 21
    versus living life, 21
Dependence on others, 54–55
Depression, 14–16, 18–19
    clinical, definition of, 14
    confusion with, 102
    medications for
        fear of dependence on, 15–16
        indications for use, 14–15, 102

neurotransmitters in, 14–15
Desire, sexual, lack of, 113–115
Diet, 95–96
Disappointment, in friend's response,
    38–39
Disclosure of cancer
    to co-workers, 72–73
    to dates, 107–110
    to new employer, 69–70
    to prospective employer, 67–68
Discontinuing treatment, 137–139
Discrimination
    legal action over, 65–67, 80
    legal protection against, 64–70
Dopamine, 15
Dwelling on experience, 9–11

E

Education, interruption in, 87–88
Emotions
    family
        communication with children,
            48–49
        consideration of older parents,
            49–50
        dismissal of recurrence possibility,
            43–44
        expectations/insensitivity of, 50–51
        sharing or understanding of patient
            feelings, 44–45
    patient/survivor
        artistic expression of, 130–131
        comparison of self with others, 9
        denial, 21
        depression, 14–16, 18–19, 102
        disappointment in friend's response,
            38–39
        dwelling on *versus* digesting
            experience, 9–11
        fear of recurrence, 6–7, 12
        feeling responsible for recurrence,
            135–136
        generalization of fear to everyday
            life, 24–25
        grieving process, 9
        hypochondria, 34–35

impatience with trivial problems, 53–54

irritability, 18–19

"letting it all out," 7–8

living with uncertainty, 29–30

mixed, at end of treatment, 4–6

post-traumatic stress disorder, 19

prognosis and, 28–30

reaction to aches and pains, 25–26

reaction to admiration for bravery, 51–52

reaction to celebrities with cancer, 33–34

reaction to compliments about appearance, 13–14

reaction to family member's results/ diagnosis, 59–61

reaction to follow-up and tests, 26–27, 32–33

reaction to friend with recurrence, 19–21

reaction to inquiries about health, 39–41

reordering of priorities, 12, 46–48

Employment. *See* Work

End of treatment
fear of recurrence after, 6–7
patient's mixed feelings about, 4–6
releasing of emotions after, 7–8

Erectile dysfunction, 111–114

Essential functions of job, 64, 82

Exercise, 28

F

Faith, loss of, 126–127

Family
change in relationship with children, 62
communication with children, 48–49
dismissal of recurrence possibility, 43–44
expectations/insensitivity of, 50–51
explanations to younger children, 55–56

feelings shared or understood by, 44–45
shielding older parents from diagnosis, 49–50
shielding survivor from other's health concerns, 61
survivor's reaction to cancer diagnosis in, 59–60

Family and Medical Leave Act (FMLA), 83

Fatigue
as after-effect, 56–58, 82, 98–99
herbal remedies for, 99
post-treatment, definition of, 82

Fears
of aches and pains, 25–26
of denial of opportunity at work, 71–72
of dependence on antidepressants, 15–16
of follow-up and tests, 26–27, 32–33
generalization to everyday life, 24–25
of others, about cancer cause, 41–43
of recurrence, 6–7, 12
of rejection, in dating situation, 109–110
of symptoms (hypochondria), 34–35

Fellow patients
comparison of self with, 9
reaction to friend with recurrence, 19–21

Fertility
adoption as alternative to, 119–121
reaction to friends', 90–91

Financial issues, 75–78, 82–83

Firing from job, 65

Five-year survival rate, 2

FMLA (Family and Medical Leave Act), 83

Focus, loss of, 101–102

Follow-up
emotional reactions to, 26–27, 32–33
frequency of, 30–32
necessity of, 30–31

recommended schedules for, 31–32
relocation and continuing of,
     102–103
Forgetfulness, 101–102
Friends
     cause of cancer inquiries from,
          41–43
     disappointment over response of,
          38–39
     insensitivity of, 45
     parenthood of, reaction to, 90–91
     pity *versus* concern from, 39–41
     problems of, patience with, 53–54
     repayment for assistance from,
          54–55
     response to after-effects, 56–58

G
Garrity, Donald, 95
Glossary, 155–157
God, anger at, 126–127
Gould, Stephen Jay, 29
Grieving process, 9

H
Hair loss, 131
"Have" *versus* "had," 3–4
Health inquiries
     from prospective employer, 68–69
     reaction to, 39–41
Health insurance
     change of job and, 77–78
     pre-existing condition and, 78
Health maintenance
     diet and, 95–96
     positive attitude and, 94
     recommendations for, 96–97
Heart damage, as late effect, 104
Herbal medicine, 99
Holland, Jimmie, 94
Home care, 138–139
Hormonal treatment
     as continuing treatment, 11
     definition of, 11
Hospice care, 138–139
Hospital, teaching, 103

Houlihan, Nancy, 104
Hypochondriac
     cancer survivor as, 34–35
     definition of, 34

I
Identity-altering experience, cancer as,
     3–4
"Imperfect" appearance, 110–111,
     117–118
Impotence, 111–114
Individual health policy, 77–78
Infertility
     adoption as alternative in, 119–121
     reaction to friends' fertility, 90–91
Information resources, 139, 141–153
Inquiries about health
     from prospective employer, 68–69
     reaction to, 39–41
Insensitivity of others, 45, 50–51
Insurance
     health, 77–78
     life, 76
Interdependence, 54–55
Irritability, 18–19

J
Job. *See* Work

K
Kleban, Roz, 134

L
Late effects, 103–104
Leflein, Tara, 55–56, 62
Legal protection/rights, 64–78, 82
"Letting it all out," 7–8
Life insurance, 76
Lung cancer, blaming patient for,
     58–59
Lung damage, as late effect, 104

M
Mammogram
     abnormal, of family member, 61
     definition of, 31

frequency of, 31
recommended screening, 96
Marriage. *See also* Spouse/partner
    changing roles/balance in, 115–116
Mather, Jane, 126
Meditation, 124
Memory loss, 101–102
Menopause, 102, 114
Mesothelioma
    definition of, 29
    Gould's experience with, 29
Metastatic disease, and survivorship,
    134–135
Moment, living in, 29–30
Mood changes
    depression, 14–16, 18–19, 102
    irritability, 18–19
Mourning, 9
Moving, and continuing follow-up,
    102–103
Moving forward, personal timetable
    for, 12

N
National Cancer Institute, 103, 134
Neuropathy, peripheral, 100–101
Neurotransmitters
    definition of, 14
    in depression, 14–15
Norepinephrine, 15
Numb sensations, 100–101
Nutrition, 95–96

O
Onassis, Jacqueline, 33
Organic foods, 95–96

P
Palliative care, 138–139
Parents, older, shielding from cancer
    diagnosis, 49–50
Peer relationships, of young survivors,
    89–90
Penile prosthesis, 112
Peripheral neuropathy, 100–101
Pity *versus* concern, 39–41

Positive changes, with cancer, 127–129
Positive thinking
    and health maintenance, 94
    "tyranny" of, 94
Post-traumatic stress disorder (PTSD),
    19
    definition of, 19
    generalization of fear in, 24–25
Post-treatment fatigue, 56–58, 82,
    98–99
Pre-existing condition
    definition of, 78
    and health insurance, 78
Priorities, reordering of, 12, 46–48
Problems of others, patience with,
    53–54
Prognosis, 28–30
Prostate specific antigen, 96
PSA blood test, 96
Psycho-motor retardation, 15
Psychotherapy group
    definition of, 16
    versus support group, 16
PTSD. *See* Post-traumatic stress
    disorder
"Put one foot in front of the other," 8

R
Radiation, definition of, 4
Radiation therapy
    end of, mixed feelings about, 4–6
    late effects of, 103–104
Reasonable accommodation, in
    workplace, 64, 79
Recurrence
    dismissal of possibility, by spouse,
        43–44
    fear of, 6–7, 12
    feeling responsible for, 135–136
    friend with, reaction to, 19–21
    statistics on, 28–30
    stress and, 97
Referral, after relocation, 102–103
Religion/spirituality, 123–131
Relocation, and continuing follow-up,
    102–103

Repayment, for help during treatment, 54–55
Resources, 139, 141–153
Resume gap, 80–81
Resuming activities/old life, 46–48

S
Sadness, 7–8, 12, 14, 19. *See also* Depression
Sarcoma, definition of, 25
"Scanitis," 32–33
Scarring, worries about, 110–111, 117–118
Screenings, recommendations for, 96
Second cancers, 104
"Self-FUL," 46
Selfishness, *versus* new priorities, 46–48
Serotonin, 15
Sexual issues, 105–121
    changing roles/balance in marriage, 115–116
    disclosure during dating, 107–110
    erectile dysfunction, 111–114
    lack of desire, 113–115
    patient–caregiver relationship and, 118–119
    relationship with spouse/partner, 106–107, 115–116, 118–119
    worry over appearance, 110–111, 117–118
"Short fuse," 18–19
Sleep problems, 14, 19, 32–33
Smoking, 27, 58–59
Social Security Disability (SSD), 82–83
Spirituality, 123–131
    cancer as "wake-up call" to, 124–125
    loss of, 126–127
Spouse/partner
    changing roles/balance with, 115–116
    dismissal of recurrence possibility by, 43–44
    feelings shared or understood by, 44–45
    patient–caregiver relationship and, 118–119

sexual relationship with, 106–107, 115–116, 118–119
Stress
    post-traumatic. *See* Post-traumatic stress disorder
    return to activities and, 97
    work and, 80
Support group(s), 16–18
    definition of, 16
    not participating in, reasons for, 17–18
    versus psychotherapy groups, 16–17
Survival statistics, 28–30
Survivorship
    defining and clarifying, 2, 134–135
    "have" *versus* "had" in, 3–4
    metastatic disease and, 134–135

T
Teaching hospital
    contacting, after relocation, 103
    definition of, 103
Temper, loss of, 18–19
Therapist, definition of, 34
Tingling sensations, 100–101
Tobacco use, 27, 58–59
Treatment
    declining further, 137–139
    end of
        fear of recurrence after, 6–7
        patient's mixed feelings about, 4–6
        releasing of emotions after, 7–8
    hormonal treatment as continuation of, 11
Trivial matters, patience with, 53–54, 73–74
"Tyranny of positive thinking," 94

U
Uncertainty, living with, 29–30
Undue hardship, on employer, 64–65

V
Vaginal changes, 114
Volunteering, 129–130
Vulnerability, feelings of, 24–25, 89–90

W

"Wake-up call," 124–125, 127–129

Weight maintenance, 28

Whittam, Beth, 86

Work

  continuing, decision on, 136–137

  disclosure after hiring, 69–70

  disclosure to co-workers, 72–73

  disclosure to prospective employer, 67–68

  documentation of concerns over, 66, 80

  essential functions in, 64, 82

  health inquiries from prospective employer, 68–69

  health insurance through, 77–78

  legal action over, 65–67, 80

  legal protection in, 64–70, 82

  loss of, during treatment, 75–76

  physical limitations at, 79

  promotions at, fear of being denied, 71–72

  reactions of co-workers, 70–71

  reasonable accommodation in, 64, 79

  resume gap and, 80–81

  return to comparable position, 65

  socializing and conversing at, 73–74

  stress in, 80

  undue hardship on employer, 64–65

Y

Yoga, 124

Young survivors

  informing doctor of childhood history, 86

  interruption in education/life, 87–88

  peer relationships of, 89–90

CPSIA information can be obtained at www.ICGtesting.com
Printed in the USA
LVOW13s2241260714

396172LV00003B/4/P